THE CAPTIVITY AND TRIUMPH OF WINNIE DAVIES

Jesus loves me, and He knows I love Him;
Love brought Him down my lost soul to redeem;
Yes, it was love made Him die on the tree;
O! it is wonderful Jesus loves me!

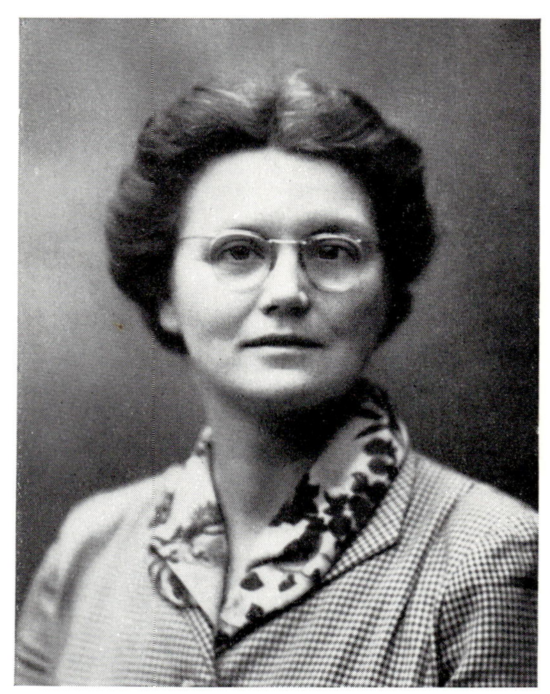

Winifred Davies
(*Killed 27th May, 1967 in North East Congo*)

THE CAPTIVITY AND TRIUMPH OF WINNIE DAVIES

by

DAVID M. DAVIES

HODDER AND STOUGHTON

First published 1968

SBN 340 04285 0

Printed in Great Britain for Hodder and Stoughton Limited,
St. Paul's House, Warwick Lane, London, E.C.4,
by Richard Clay (The Chaucer Press), Ltd., Bungay, Suffolk

ACKNOWLEDGEMENTS

I am happy to acknowledge my indebtedness to many friends who have freely helped me with typing, giving information and lending letters and photographs.

In particular I must mention Mr Len Moules, Mr and Mrs Robert Butters (for the use of their diary), Pastor Alieni Paul, Dr Helen Roseveare, Father Alphons Strijbosch, Mr Norman P. Grubb for details concerning Zamu the lame evangelist, and Miss Mary Endersbee for her invaluable help in editing the manuscript.

Lutterworth Press very kindly gave me permission to use material on the life of Mrs Edith Moules from their publication *Mighty Through God* by Norman P. Grubb.

Royalties from this book go to help further the work of the Worldwide Evangelization Crusade.

DAVID M. DAVIES

INTRODUCTION

A few moments ago I finished reading this manuscript and with the string-tied pages still in my lap, I wish to say first of all, "Don't read this book unless you really want to!" This book is dynamite. What could you expect when it was written surrounded by prayer, and when the "dynamos" of the Spirit had touched the mind of the writer? The text between these covers has the potential to halt the course of your life and revolutionize it.

What I mean is this. There is a lot of easy and ignorant talk these days concerning the ultimate purpose of life, and the standards by which to live this neo-existence. This produces an aimless, drifting, frustrated, codeless society. Winnie Davies found the ultimate purpose of life and enjoyed it. I'll say that again and correct my mistake. Winnie Davies found the ultimate purpose of life and enjoyed *Him.*

Jesus Christ dominated her life. He brought meaning into living by a glorious consciousness of forgiveness and love as shown to her in His Cross. She knew God wanted her for Himself and for His purpose. She accepted that divine commission and gave herself completely and utterly to His enabling. His inward presence fulfilling that objective. She glorified her Saviour by her life – and by her death.

The standards she lived by were down-to-earth interpretations of God's mandate for life as read in the Scriptures. She didn't dodge issues by "spiritualizing" them when those issues demanded practical expressions of obedience.

Yet Winnie was still very much a human being in spite of all that. She was a strong personality of sterling character. The former could at times create a difficult situation for her God-appointed leaders in the Fellowship. Courses of action were supported by an adamant determination to pursue them, often against wise counselling for adjustment in time or method. It never reached the point of disobedience – she was far too loyal for that – but she knew how to put pressure into her reasoning.

So this book has a punch, and it hits where it hurts. You are going to do exactly what I have done – sit back and admit that the ease and softness of modern life has eaten like a cancer into the sinew and fibre of my life – whether it be physical or spiritual, or both. By Winnie's standard we are soft, and we men will find it hurts the more.

The book does not leave us in despondency. Winnie is constantly telling us where she found the essential resources. Don't read this book unless you are prepared to finish it on your knees.

LEN MOULES
International Secretary,
Worldwide Evangelization Crusade,
Bulstrode, Gerrards Cross, Bucks.

CONTENTS

ILLUSTRATIONS

PROLOGUE

"Constantly under the supervision of a Simba guard armed with a spear, Winifred Davies and Father Alphons Strijbosch were forced, barefoot, to draw water and to gather firewood for the new regime . . .

"Miss Davies continued her maternity work with 'extreme devotion' to the end and served as midwife to the wife of a Simba forty-eight hours before her death. She unsparingly nursed even her captors.

"For the last three days of forced march to flee from the approaching National Army, neither Miss Davies nor the priest had anything to eat. The priest, overcome with faintness, fell twice . . . He lost the way. Suddenly he saw Miss Davies lying on her back, peacefully, as though resting.

"She does not move. She is dead.

"Too weak to keep up with the flight she had fallen . . . Wounds on the forehead and throat and the blood still fresh . . . She could not have been dead more than fifteen minutes.

"Five hundred yards further on three soldiers appeared from the undergrowth. They raised their guns. Thinking his end had come Father Strijbosch crossed himself, threw up his arms and waited for the shots.

" 'Halt! Are you the Roman Catholic priest?'

" 'Yes, I am.'

" 'We are National Army soldiers. You are liberated!' "

Le Courrier d'Afrique
(June 12th 1967)

"It will take more than a jungle, more than a bullet, more than blind savagery, to still the inspiration which flowed from her great heart."

The People
(June 11th 1967)

THE CAPTIVITY AND TRIUMPH OF WINNIE DAVIES

Winifred Davies, constrained by the compassion of Christ, gave herself for twenty-one years without restraint for the good of the Congolese people. On her lonely mission station, at the end of a desperately treacherous road, in one of the densest spots of the great Ituri forest, she built her hospital, the only maternity unit within a hundred miles.

The undiscriminating, savage Simba rebels took her captive and held her for thirty-three months.

The Congolese Christians loved her. They willingly suffered to protect her. Alieni Paul was trussed and hung up in a tree, released, beaten and again hung up and left hanging for hours; then empty cartridge shells were rammed over his fingers – because of his efforts to help her. He is still alive and is glad that he suffered in his gallant attempts.

Reports of Winnie's Christian life among the Simbas serve to still the "why" in the hearts of those who prayed for her deliverance. Across her thirty-three months of privation, hunger and terror can be written the words of another who suffered for the sake of the gospel: "The things which happened unto me have fallen out rather unto the furtherance of the gospel" (Paul in Philippians 1:12).

What was said of Isabel Kuhn can also be said of Winnie Davies: "Hers was not the tragedy of a premature death but the triumph of a fulfilled ministry." (*One Vision Only* by Carolyn Canfield, CIM).

1

FROM COEDPOETH TO LIVERPOOL

"Matron, I want to make a confession."

Matron studied the open, earnest face of Nurse Winifred Davies with some surprise. Wasn't this the timid Welsh girl who had joined the Probationers Training School some month previously?

"I've been . . . I've been helping myself to food from the kitchens, you see. Usually on night duty – because we were hungry. I'm very sorry, Matron, and I want to repay the hospital for what I've taken."

Nurse Davies paused, swallowed, then rushed on.

"You see, I've become a Christian and I want to make amends. I would like to make a fresh start if I may, please."

. . .

Bootle General Hospital may have had some notable trainee nurses through its PTS classes, but few young student nurses will have stepped into Matron's office to make a similar statement. And few would have expected it from Winifred Davies.

Born on November 30th 1915, the second child of a master watchmaker at Coedpoeth, some four miles from Wrexham, her upbringing produced a timid though friendly nineteen year old launching on a nursing career with no particular religious intent.

As she made friends at the hospital her love for her home and its surroundings was most evident in her conversation. Often she mentioned her "Mama", Alice Davies, who had lavished affection on the three of them, Leslie, Winnie and Dorothy;

and her "Dada", Howell Davies, who worked hard and long hours for little money but had made the home a happy one despite few luxuries. Born in Coedpoeth on January 26th 1886, the son of a collier in the North Wales coalfield, Howell Davies understood only too well the uncertainties and dangers faced by his customers, many of them miners too. His father-in-law was also a miner, and this family background made him generous towards those who could not always afford to give him the full payment for his work.

But instead of luxuries in the home, joy was found in simpler things like baking, for instance, which was Winnie's great delight. She loved to "help" her mother with the cooking.

"There's flour from one end of the house to the other!" Mrs Davies would exclaim when Winnie had finished and disappeared to look after a neighbour's baby, managing to leave every dish in the house dirty!

Music was another source of enjoyment to the family. Winnie was encouraged to learn the piano and gladly walked eight miles for lessons at Tan-y-fron. She made good progress, developing a taste for the classic composers.

Then there were outings and picnics, a favourite entertainment for Leslie and Dorothy as well. Sugar butty sandwiches were the main course and a place about a quarter of a mile from home the best-loved spot. Winnie could also recall when they had been more adventurous and had walked six miles just for the joy of the train ride back – for the princely sum of a penny each!

From her earliest days Winnie was happier with people than with books. Her education at Penygelli Junior and Penygelli Central Schools had never enthralled her or produced more than average results. She would rush in from school, fling her satchel in the corner and gulp down her tea.

"Just going to mind Mrs Jones' baby, Mama," or "Old Miss Morris wants me to help her with her garden," she would explain, as she kissed her mother and rushed out again.

When she left school at sixteen her first job was as a dentist's clerk in Wrexham. Though she enjoyed having some money to spend on clothes, after two years the lack of prospects for the future made her restless. Nursing had a growing appeal for her and she wrote to a friend, Martha Eluned Jones, for advice. Martha Eluned had been accepted as a student nurse in a hospital in Tooting, and her reply was certainly realistic.

"Nursing is a hard life with long hours and neither time nor money for recreation," she wrote. "You must make up your own mind."

An incident in September 1934 may have helped Winnie to make her decision. At 2 am on the morning of September 22nd 1934 at Gresford Colliery just outside Wrexham, an explosion followed by fire destroyed one shaft of the mine, killing 265 men, three of them rescuers. Only eleven bodies were recovered before the shaft was sealed off, and a lengthy enquiry started. The report of this enquiry was debated in the House of Commons and measures were taken to prevent a similar occurrence. It was the worst disaster in the history of British coalmining.

The whole country was shaken by this tragedy, while hardly a home in the immediate district around Gresford was left untouched by some personal loss of relative or friend. Winnie saw, perhaps for the first time, what compassion could do in the face of human grief and need. Her love of people coupled with the desire to help them spurred her on to apply to Bootle General Hospital for training, and she was accepted.

It was probable that the drab streets of Bootle awakened nostalgic memories of Coedpoeth and its scenery in Winnie, for her home-sickness, when she began her training on April 7th 1935, was hard to bear.

From her home set on the slopes of Esclusham Mountain she had been able to see a great panorama of open country, taking in seven counties. Despite the inevitable pithead scenery of the nearby coalfields, the distant mountains and hills drew her eyes across the expanse of fields and valleys. Looking east she could see the Dee valley, with the meandering river deeply embedded in its green pastureland. Beyond lay the flat Cheshire plain stretching away towards the Pennines, and in the foreground lay Wrexham, the nearest big town, with St Giles's parish church spire as its landmark.

Turning her eyes south, the hills of Shropshire rolled away into Merionethshire and the lowlands of Staffordshire. Her own county of Denbighshire climbed away to the west, but the mountains hid the higher ranges of Snowdon and Caernarvonshire from her view. Instead the Clwyd range with its highest peak, Moel Fammau, drew her gaze to Flintshire and down to the Dee estuary. Then northwards across Cheshire she could just see the haze and smoke of Liverpool and the Lancashire mills.

As she travelled the forty-odd miles from Coedpoeth to Liverpool, her trepidation at leaving her beloved Coedpoeth was matched by a determination to make a success of nursing. She did not realize that her journey was to mean more than a change of scenery; it was to mean a change of heart also.

. . .

"Scott! Scott! Look, here's a parcel from home. Do open it quickly now. It will be another cake and I love your mother's cake, you know I do."

Winnie dumped the parcel in Nurse Margaret Scott's hands expectantly. Her appetite, which was so often her undoing, was known to her friend (now Mrs Margaret Stephenson), who remembers: "I got very little of my own fruit cakes!"

Perhaps this explains why, when food was short and Winnie was on night duty, she often climbed into the pantry through a small window to pilfer food for her fellow nurses. Her friendliness and readiness to help others were always evident once she had overcome the timidity that her sheltered background had given her, and she soon became, in her own words, "a worldly young nurse". She dashed everywhere, cloak and cap awry and swearing with the best of them, although boy friends and dancing were not in her line.

But for all her apparent vivacity a deep dissatisfaction was beginning to trouble her during those years of training. She had gone with a friend to a meeting of the Nurses' Christian Fellowship held in the hospital, and she had also attended meetings at Emmanuel Hall, a nearby mission. For the first time in her life she was facing the claims of Jesus Christ and it shook her deeply.

She turned the problem over and over in her mind. From her childhood she could remember her parents attending church. Howell Davies attended the Welsh Wesleyan church but Alice, being of Danish descent, knew no Welsh and attended the English church of St Tudfil in Coedpoeth. It was at St Tudfil's that Winnie had been christened and later confirmed, and she was soon active in the church as a Sunday school teacher and worker in the Girls' Friendly Society. Wasn't all this a sure sign that she was a Christian? She had been faithful to her Church and when others had spoken unkindly of it she had defended it strongly. Why, even now she said her prayers sporadically and, from a sense of duty, read bits of the Bible, though she had to admit she found it hard to understand and uninteresting. Yet God and Jesus Christ seemed strangers to her, while others appeared to know and love them personally.

Troubled over these perplexities and her own shortcomings she slept badly, searching for peace of mind. Slowly it became clear to her that Jesus Christ had died in order to make possible the forgiveness of her past wrongs. He had died to give her peace with God and bring her into his family. She had known these facts for years but suddenly it came home to her: Jesus had died for *her*.

It was the love of Christ that won her heart; everything else took second place. With no reservations she gave herself to Him. His love and the wonder of His sacrifice for her became her great theme and drew from her the response, often repeated then and later: "I love Jesus Christ with every fibre of my being."

No particular date or experience seems to be connected with this "change of heart" but Winnie, with characteristic vigour soon made her new position known to her friends and colleagues.

Not only was Matron faced by a determined Winnie seeking to make restitution, but the rest of her group knew something had happened. Amidst the clamour of the nurses' dining room, where each nurse was making an all-out effort to eat as much as possible in the shortest space of time, Winnie would pause to bow her head to thank God for her food. Her fellow nurses never forgot the day she raised her head from saying grace as a servant was passing a plate of soup. Head and plate met with a thud and Winnie got the contents over her uniform, but treated it as a great joke!

It was this radiance and buoyancy of spirit that made itself felt in those grim days when the threat of war was rapidly becoming reality. Winnie was quick to appraise a situation and to act, usually with an infectious smile or laugh, and her guilelessness when speaking about her faith seldom stirred up abuse. A typical instance was when she challenged a Liverpool bus conductor about his blasphemous language, with a firm "It's my Saviour you're talking about."

She spent time talking and praying with her friends in the hospital. Nurse Margaret Oldfield was one of these: "I remember thinking how kind her eyes were. She talked to me about my sin and my need of a saviour. Probably my ignorant answers prompted her to ask whether I believed in the whole of the Bible. I replied 'Of course not! Do you?' We then knelt down and Winnie prayed. A few weeks later another nurse, who had been converted through Winnie, helped me to accept the Lord as my Saviour."

Winnie had found a new purpose and meaning in life and she described this later. "I began to see the meaning of the hymns we used to sing and they seemed so beautiful and so marvellous that I felt the hymn-book must have been altered! But the change was not in the book but in me. I also wondered what I used to teach my Sunday School children. Often I read portions of the Bible to them but I did not know the Saviour in those days."

In her nursing a new dedication became apparent. Margaret

Stephenson recalls, "Winnie was not in any sense a dedicated nurse until she became a senior, and she had always been terrified of theatre work. Yet she became a good theatre nurse and began talking about tropical medicine and wishing she was clever enough to become a doctor. It was at this time she made up her mind to take all the certificates that would help her become as proficient as possible."

So, her course at Bootle General Hospital finished, in August 1938 Winnie went on to Smithdown Road Hospital and then the Fazakerly Isolation Hospital. She qualified as a State Registered Nurse and as a midwife – receiving her SCM on May 23rd 1939 – and then as a State Registered Fever Nurse.

During these years her rare quality of tenderness and compassion for suffering grew, when it might well have diminished. A friend remembers: "I became seriously ill and was taken to hospital. Winnie was present when I was X-rayed and sat with me after my admission to the ward. To my surprise I noticed that she was crying. On enquiring the reason I found her to be deeply affected by the somewhat 'ungentle' handling of me during the X-ray examinations. Doubtless her soft heart exaggerated things, for I have no memory of any extra pain caused at that time. Then she said, 'Oh, dear Miss Dann, I do wish we could change places and that I could bear the pain instead of you."

These qualifications, in nursing and in compassion, were all-important to Winnie's future work, but the only hint we have of her own intentions at that time are her words spoken at a later date: "I asked the Lord Jesus to save me; then I asked Him to please forgive my sins and come to live in my heart through His Spirit. About six months later I asked Him to fill me with His mighty Holy Spirit, and as soon as I asked Him to do this I told my friends that I would be willing to go to the mission field and serve Him amongst the lepers if He wanted me to do so. So I started seeking God's will for my life."

God had work for her to do; but not knowing exactly what or where, Winnie decided she would benefit from some Bible college training. She applied to Emmanuel Bible College in Birkenhead, just a ferry-ride across the River Mersey from the Pier Head, Liverpool. She was accepted and began a three-year course there in 1941 as the war was entering its third year and the bombing of Merseyside was to become a nightly ordeal.

2

BIRKENHEAD, WEC AND WAITING

From the start of her course at Emmanuel Bible College Winnie was liked by her fellow students. She bubbled over with joy, entering into everything with zest and often becoming spokeswoman for the others. She proved herself a natural leader and was chosen as head student for part of her course.

Even in the college atmosphere of firm spiritual discipline she was always ready for a laugh. It was wartime so food was short, which may explain why Winnie, when laying the tables for lunch and seeing dessert spoons, was heard to exclaim, "Praise the Lord, there's pudding today!"

Margaret Oldfield, her friend from nursing days, came to visit her at college and remembers how Winnie reacted on seeing her manner of dress. Margaret liked dressing fashionably and using make-up, but went to Emmanuel to meet Winnie dressed "as I thought a Christian ought to dress! When Winnie caught sight of me she took me aside and gave me one of her precious lectures. 'Now, don't you do what I did when I was first saved. I thought I had to wear black stockings, flat-heeled shoes and my hair tied back as tightly as possible. On top of that I went around looking miserable!' Dear Winnie! Someone must have given her the same lecture because her face was seldom anything but radiant."

A close friend at college was Frances Linklater (now Mrs Lyons), who recalls another typical incident. "For one of the many two-hour periods in the prayer room, it was my turn to spend the session with Winnie. As we walked out of the prayer room along the landing to the stairs Winnie gripped my arm and exclaimed, 'Oh Frances, isn't the Lord wonderful! I am so utterly thrilled with Him I feel I could slide down the banister.' She promptly did so, arriving at the bottom just as Mr Drysdale, the Principal, came out of the dining room! Maybe only ex-students can appreciate the horror of that moment!"

On a more serious level Winnie constantly showed her love for people. On Saturday evenings the students went "pubbing". They visited local public houses, offering the college magazine for sale and talking about their faith with those who would listen. Frances says, "I can see Winnie now, leaning on a table in a smoke-filled beer lounge and speaking straightforwardly to the drinking, laughing and sometimes mocking women. Time after time I saw her deep sincerity completely win their attention. Often there were tears as they listened to her speak of her own experience. Then she would pray with them and urge them to take Christ as their Saviour, leaving them with a warm 'God bless you. I shall pray for you'.

"It was the same in open air meetings. Winnie would stand on the box and tell the crowd what Jesus meant to her. In the homes of the poor folk on Merseyside and in the hospital visitation Winnie was always telling someone of her Saviour."

Frances remembers most vividly the night she experienced Winnie's simple and practical concern for herself. "It was towards the end of term and I was extremely tired. I was low in spirit and weeping beside my bed, when Winnie came in asking what was wrong. I poured out my problem, telling her that I would have to leave college at once as I was not fit to be there as a student. I was much too sinful and the Lord had told me how bad I was.

"Winnie listened patiently until I finished and then said in a firm voice: 'That is the voice of Satan and you should know by now he is a liar. Stop talking any more. Get into bed and go to sleep.' I said I couldn't sleep; I had tried in vain but it was no good. Winnie knelt down and prayed, laying hands on me and telling Satan, in Jesus' name, to leave me alone. Then she told me to get into bed, adding, 'If the Lord sends sleep, that will be the end of the matter. If not, perhaps the Lord is speaking to you and we must think again.' I was asleep in five minutes and awoke in the morning feeling on top of the world."

Frances adds, "But Winnie could sometimes be forceful, even domineering. As senior student she was very much in command of us, and woe betide anyone who tried to cross her. On one occasion we were all sitting at the table studying and I was very tired. Winnie noticed and wrote a little note to me: 'Frances, go off to bed.' As I felt this would be wrong at study time I sent a little note back saying so. Winnie, using her most commanding tone, exclaimed loudly so that everyone could hear: 'Sister Linklater, *do as you're told*!' I knew I had to go; I just dared not argue any further!"

Frances and Winnie shared a dormitory and it was then that Winnie discovered, at last, God's purpose for her future. Frances had spent half a night in prayer and was returning to the room in the early hours of the morning. "As far as I was aware all the other students were asleep. But as I tiptoed softly in I heard someone sobbing. I listened and realized the sobs came from Winnie's bed. Shining my torch I saw her kneeling figure shaking with sobs, her head buried in her hands.

"I left her alone at first but then decided to go and offer help, for she did seem to be greatly distressed. To my question she replied, 'Oh Frances, it's come. The Lord has called me to the Lepers and I have to go to the Congo.'

"I really couldn't understand why she was so upset. To me it was the most wonderful thing to be called to serve God in Africa. Winnie agreed with me, but she was concerned for her mother. 'I think it will kill her,' she said, 'and it may mean death for me. But that doesn't matter. It is my poor mother; I know it will break her heart.' "

But Winnie knew she had heard God's voice and she began to pray, not only for her mother but to know what the next step should be. As her course drew to its close she became certain that the Worldwide Evangelization Crusade was the missionary society to which she should apply on leaving college.

Looking back over her three years at college, Winnie had to admit she had learnt some hard lessons. She had done well at her studies, but the most valuable lesson was in the art of practical, holy living: learning to live at close quarters with other people; learning to become a disciple through being disciplined.

One of the first things that had impressed her as she was shown round the main building was the painted motto which reads, "I refuse to be discouraged: I will only praise." Another picture which daily challenged her bore the words, "Go through." The need for this spirit of perseverance was obviously close to the heart of the Principal, the late Pastor J. D. Drysdale. Winnie remembered the day he had stood looking at this large picture depicting the Christians of the early Church being thrown to the lions in the arena. He turned to the group of students behind him and said, "The early believers were tested. The days of persecution may return. Remember those words, 'Go through.' Can you go through? Do you have that spirit?"

His words meant a great deal to her then and in the future. As she left the college her heartfelt desire for "that spirit" was summed up in her two favourite verses from the Bible: "Be thou faithful unto death" (Rev. 2 : 10) and "Christ shall be magnified in my body, whether it be by life, or by death" (Phil. 1 : 20).

. . .

It was August 1944 when Winnie applied to the Worldwide Evangelization Crusade for missionary work in the Congo. Her application involved her in a stay at the headquarters of the mission in south-east London.

The headquarters were in Highland Road, Gipsy Hill, a short distance from the old Crystal Palace. Numbers 17 and 19 were stamped with history, for this was where WEC was born; where the founders, Mr and Mrs C. T. Studd, had lived; and it was from there that C. T. Studd had left to pioneer and spend the remainder of his life in the Congo. On the plot of Number 17, a building which had been a cats' home was converted into suitable business offices, deputation department, equipment rooms and dormitories; in front of this building a fine, large, modern hostel was built. On the opposite side of the road, WEC also owned two old but well-built houses, Numbers 32 and 34. These housed the staff, the candidates, the Leper and Medical Crusade workers and offices, and the laundry. The whole place was always humming with activity as daily arrivals and departures took place. (The WEC headquarters have now moved to a large country house at Gerrards Cross.)

Winnie entered into the busy life at Highland Road with enthusiasm. During her time there she studied the principles and literature of the WEC, finding in particular that the biography of C. T. Studd, the founder of the mission, thrilled her. Most of all his motto "If Jesus Christ be God and died for me, then no sacrifice can be too great for me to make for Him" found a ready echo in her own heart and encouraged her in the days ahead.

After several interviews she was accepted as a candidate, but her departure was delayed by war restrictions. In fact the bombing was so bad that part of the WEC personnel had to leave London, and Winnie seized the opportunity to go to the Continent to study French for some months, knowing that the language would be one she would have to use in the Congo.

David and Chrissie Batchelor, with whom she stayed while abroad, remember her "personal charm and indomitable purpose in life. The thing that impressed us most of all was her conception of true holiness. She had been to Emmanuel Bible College and had seen and experienced what holiness means. And for her it meant being holy right down to the smallest things and a humbling of herself in confession to others. Winnie wanted nothing to be between her and her Lord, and she was so joyful. How her face used to light up with a lovely smile as she talked. Her joy in the Lord was really infectious."

Delay followed delay, and June 1945 found Winnie at the WEC Conference at Llandudno – not so far from her home – in North Wales. It was to provide further confirmation of her decision to apply for work in the Congo. Although she was accepted by the mission, her future destination was still unsure; but as she listened to Mrs Edith Moules, pioneer of much of the medical work in the Congo, she felt increasingly sure that God's future work for her lay there.

Mrs Moules was describing the work of the dispensary she had set up, with its three hundred patients gathering in the evening for treatment: ". . . Suddenly, at the back of them all – he had been standing there unobserved for a while – I saw a leper. I had seen lepers before, but this man was terribly mutilated. He was led by a small boy and was almost naked. His toes and fingers were gone; his feet swollen. He had no nose and he was dribbling from his lipless mouth, down over his bare body. Both he and the child looked travel-stained and hungry. I suddenly became contagion-conscious. I did not want to touch that man and I said to myself, 'Oh, we cannot have a leper here. Whatever shall I do?'

"I looked at him every now and again and wondered what I should say to him. Finally, when everybody had gone, he hobbled around and the small boy looked up wistfully into my face and said, 'We have come to come.'

" 'Well, where have you come from?'

" 'The other side of Poko.' Nearly a hundred miles! More than eighty miles through the forest he had walked with feet like that, swollen to bursting point. It must have taken them days and days.

"That was the moral issue I had to face. The man needed help. He needed outward help as do many others. It is no use thinking that we can go out and preach the gospel and shut our eyes to facts. We cannot have that hard heart which says, 'I must not look at the suffering of people. I must not look at their aches and worries. I have come just to be an evangelist.' I could have done that with leanness to my soul. I could have said, as I did say to God, 'I came here to evangelize' . . . but here was I up against my problem. The little boy said, 'We have come to come,' and I had no leper hospital and no intention of building one or of starting a leper work. I had not even thought about it. All my plans were made, and they did not include the lepers. What was I going to do?"

Mrs Moules went on to tell how the battle raged within her for four days until it was "finally fought out". She had given the couple an old tumbledown shack and food, but it was the story of the Good Samaritan that brought vividly to her mind the challenge of loving her neighbour as herself. "It was not until I realized that the leper was *my* neighbour that I could get peace", and the decision was made to open a leprosy centre at Nebobongo.

At the close of the address Mrs Moules mentioned the need for a fully qualified nurse at this hospital in Nebobongo in north-east Congo, to take over the maternity work which she herself had left. The leper work was catered for, but the general medical work needed the supervision of a trained nurse and the maternity work had ceased on her departure.

Deeply challenged by Mrs Moule's frankness and knowing her training fitted her for the work, Winnie offered herself specifically for the post at Nebobongo. An interview was arranged with Mrs Moules and Winnie attended with some trepidation. "I do feel nervous about going to see Mrs Moules," she confided to a friend. "I feel too unworthy to even offer for such a great work. Do you think she will accept me?"

She need not have feared. Edith Moules talked long and seriously with her. They prayed together, then she gladly accepted Winnie's offer for Nebobongo. With a deeper assurance than ever that God had called her to help the people of Congo, Winnie determined to serve God and the Congolese with all her powers. There was to be no turning back.

But it was to be more than a year before she could leave for the Congo – a year of waiting and speaking at missionary meetings. Winnie accepted many invitations to speak, and Margaret Coleman who was with her remembers, "Winnie was an acceptable speaker, winsome and at the same time challenging. One important meeting for some reason was very flat and heavy. Seasoned workers failed to get any vital message across but Winnie, the missionary candidate, had God's message and blessed many with it."

The secret of Winnie's winsome and powerful preaching was not in her natural ability. Rather it was the fruit of her complete devotion to Christ and her absolute trust in the Spirit of God to help her to deliver a message.

Once she was challenged about this. She was booked to speak at two meetings. On the way home after the first she was asked if she had been filled with the Holy Spirit. Without hesitation and almost emphatically she replied, "Yes, I have." She was then asked if this "filling" had been accompanied by certain manifestations and she gave a negative reply. "Then," remonstrated her friend, "do not dare to go to the mission field till you have had this experience, or no souls will be won and you will return an empty failure."

Although Winnie was sympathetic towards her friend's belief and experience she could not see that the winning of souls was dependent on an experience. She was greatly upset by the conversation and did not want to go to the second meeting the following night. But she spent time in prayer and quietly sorting out the problem, and when the time came to leave for the meeting she was ready; happy to go and trusting that the Lord would make her a blessing. That night she spoke simply but with much power. Two members of the congregation heard, in her message, the voice of God. One was a person who had resisted the Lord for some time and finally yielded in faith to Him. The other was a backslider who found his faith restored. Winnie proved the genuineness of her sanctification with this evidence of God's power working through her.

At a ministers' retreat at St Helens, Lancashire, in 1945 the expected missionary speaker was ill and only his wife and Winnie could attend. Olive Moore describes the retreat: "On arrival there was great consternation because there were only two women and *no* man for a minsters' gathering! There was nothing else for it but to do the best we could. Winnie was to give her testimony and the story of her call and I was to speak on the Congo.

"Winnie spoke with such power that the men were stirred to attention. She finished her testimony, as she did on a number of occasions, with the words 'I love the Lord with all my heart because He has done so much for me, and I want to serve Him with every fibre of my being.' It did not seem to matter after that, that two mere women had come to address their meeting!"

For about six months of that year of waiting Winnie stayed at the newly opened Welsh WEC headquarters on Mount Pleasant Hill, Swansea, for which Bill and Ena Pethybridge were responsible. They remember her stay with gratitude. "Although Winnie was so obviously 'filled with the Spirit' she was very far from being 'so heavenly-minded as to be of no earthly use'! She would buckle into any practical jobs with great gusto, doing them joyfully and efficiently. As we had moved into an old house recently after bomb damage, there was much practical work to be done and we were most grateful for the help she gave."

During her stay in Swansea, Winnie for the first time received financial help in answer to prayer. All accepted candidates were to look to God alone for the supply of their equipment and passage money, with no promise of help from the mission. Winnie was faced with a need of £100 to complete her passage expenses. True to the principle of the WEC she made her need known to God alone. Bill and Ena remember that "after much prayer she was sure the money would come, believing the verse Mark 11 : 24 – 'What things soever ye desire, when ye pray, believe that ye receive them, and ye shall have them.' "

Mrs Rogers, who also lived at the headquarters, continues the story: "A few days later we found a bulky envelope pushed inside the front door with 'Miss Winnie Davies' written on it. Winnie was away at meetings around Glamorganshire and Carmarthenshire for many days, and we felt anxious about this letter lying on the dresser without acknowledgement. Then a wire came asking if the letter had been received. What should we do? The next moment the door opened and Winnie came in.

When she opened the envelope there was nothing in it except fifty £1 notes! She left Swansea a few days later."

The morning she left Swansea for her final preparations in London Mrs Rogers remembers her coming into their bedroom with tears streaming down her face. "I've come to say goodbye," she said, putting her arms around husband and wife and adding, "Lord, I'm not sufficient." But she soon found comfort in the verse "our sufficiency is of God" (2 Cor. 3 : 5) and flung herself into the business of collecting her luggage together for her sailing date on July 25th.

Back in London the time seemed to fly. Buying equipment, packing, speaking at the last few meetings and one or two visits home to her beloved family and friends in Coedpoeth filled her days.

One of her visits home coincided with that of a relative from overseas and a spontaneous party was the result. Winnie entered into the fun with obvious enjoyment, but a serious note was struck when a friend's question voiced the feelings of many.

"Is it safe for you to go to Congo?" she was asked. To go to Africa and live with lepers seemed like going to the end of the earth to throw one's life away. Was it really necessary? Winnie's answer revealed that her future safety did not concern her at all. "God has told me to go," she replied, as if all the dangers ahead were thus nullified.

But for all her confidence in God it was no easy matter to leave her home and family, and Winnie, who hated saying goodbye at the best of times, had a hard time ahead.

Her father was in favour of her decision to go, and encouraged her, but her mother found the parting very painful. Many months before when she had shared her concern for her mother with Frances Linklater at Emmanuel, she had also asked other friends to pray that her mother would let her go gladly. Two such friends were Tom and Sarah Evans of Swansea. On her last visit to them before sailing, Winnie arrived beaming and waving a letter.

"Listen, wonderful news! I had this letter from my mother

this morning and she says, 'My angel, I have given you to the lepers.' " There were tears of gratitude for answered prayer on that occasion and there were tears of human sorrow when the moment of parting for mother and daughter came. But Winnie maintained: "I have to obey the One above." She loved her parents deeply but the One who had died for her held the prior claim on her life.

3

NEBOBONGO AT LAST

"I hope Winnie will be like an atom bomb for God in the Congo!" said Howell Davies, turning to the group of missionary headquarters staff and friends gathered at Victoria to see Winnie off. It was 25th July, 1946 and the Southampton train carrying Winnie was fast dwindling to a speck as it gathered speed.

The boat journey from Southampton to Matadi on the west coast of Africa was uneventful. Once she was through the customs at the port, Winnie took a train to Leopoldville (now Kinshasa) and there caught a slow steamer up the Congo River to Stanleyville (now Kisangani). The trip took a week, and after this slow progress Winnie was delighted to find Frank Cripps and the mission truck awaiting her at Stanleyville. The rest of the three hundred mile journey overland was a bone-shaking experience but well worth the tumultuous welcome she received on arriving at Wamba mission station, where she was to stay for a short period.

As she travelled inland Winnie was enchanted with all she saw and determined not to miss anything. From the train she had picked out many small villages of mud houses roofed with grass or leaves, and she loved the little naked "totos" running and playing around the doorways. As they drove along the Route Ituri the dense forest suddenly seemed to close around them, drenching the road with green shadows. Often the road crossed rivers by bridges, fords or ferries, including the ferry at Ngayu. Winnie couldn't bear to sit in the cab in the stifling heat and miss all the excitement while they waited their turn to cross. Despite Frank's warnings about bites from the many riverside flies Winnie got out and stood watching the men handling the planks and ferry. When she climbed back into the cab she had to confess she had been severely bitten, but her mounting excitement at nearing her destination soon made her forget her stings.

At last the truck pulled into Wamba mission station. All the five hundred school children, dressed in their best clothes or uniforms, marched past singing to the accompaniment of a deafening assembly of cornets, bugles and drums. And from every direction workers and local Christians came streaming across the compound to greet Winnie with a welcoming handshake. For days her hand was wrung until it was limp. The Congolese came, it seemed at least ten times a day, to shake hands and say *Jambo Mademoiselle* for the joy (or was it the fun?) of hearing her first stumbling attempts at returning their greeting with *Jambo sana.*

Not only did the people give her intense joy; the picturesque scenery of the compound thrilled her too – the red roads and paths crossing green lawns, the tall, graceful palm trees shading the buildings of mud and home-made red brick, and most of all the flowers with their brilliant colours. Roses, gladioli, frangipani, plumbago bushes, a fine arch of "golden chain" at the entrance to the main mission house and beautiful hedges of hibiscus revealed the care of the missionaries and their helpers. The overall effect made Winnie feel she had stepped into dreamland.

But any dreamlike qualities in her arrival were soon dispelled. Her stings and bites were developing into an intensely painful skin infection. The local doctor was called to give her an injection, but her body reacted against it. He tried something else, and again the reaction was severe. This continued until the doctor did not know what else to do and her hands, arms and legs were completely covered with bandages. The problem seemed insurmountable and there was even talk of her being returned home. Winnie was so disturbed by this suggestion that she asked the field leader who was at Wamba, Mr Jack Scholes, if she could be anointed and prayed for. Jack Scholes agreed and the next day, as there was a communion service, Winnie was anointed before all the people and they prayed for her recovery, trusting the Lord to do a work of healing. It was remarkable that within a week she was perfectly well again.

During this gruelling experience Winnie never lost her confidence that God had called her to Congo, and this enabled her to keep smiling despite the pain. Perhaps it was this disposition which led Jack Scholes to choose for her the Swahili name *Mama Furaha* (locally pronounced "Foo-rah," with the accent on the last syllable). The English equivalent would be "Mother Joy"; she could not have been given a better name, for the Congolese, always quick to appraise character and give an appropriate name in their own tribal language, were pleased with the choice and never changed it. This saved Winnie the embarrassment some of her colleagues faced when they learnt the tribal language and discovered what their "nickname" really meant! Invariably the name was a true summary of their character and not necessarily very flattering!

As Winnie recovered from the effects of her allergy she made a start on her language study. From Wamba she was moved to Ibambi, the headquarters station some sixty miles north; there she was, at last, allocated to Nebobongo, the medical centre that Edith Moules had so vividly described at Llandudno. Nebobongo was about eight miles north of Ibambi, and she was to be with Will and Rhodie Dawn. At the centre, with its leper, general medical and maternity work founded by Percy and Edith Moules, Arthur Scott had wonderfully filled the gap created by the absence of Mrs Moules, (following the death of her husband). He was in charge of the actual leper work on the compound, and supervised five leper settlements in the district. Will and Rhodie were responsible for the clean children of leper parents and the general administration of the compound. At that time there were about sixty-four untainted children and ten babies "on the bottle".

In all there were about 1,300 lepers under direct supervision when Winnie arrived in 1946, and the work was most encouraging from every point of view. Young men and women were being trained for responsible positions. Some, trained as artisans, were training others; there were leper brick-makers, builders, carpenters and a tailor. The peanut crop was yielding about ten tons a year and the rice plantations gave a surplus of two tons. Furthermore, a Bible school had just been started to train young Christian lepers in Bible knowledge.

The great day arrived when Jack Scholes drove Winnie to Nebobongo. As they motored along she was delighted at the welcome they received from the Africans who recognized the mission car, and she tried to return their shouted greetings. The villages they passed were clean and well kept, each surrounded by its cotton gardens, cluster of coffee trees, plantains and tall palm trees. Then, after passing the Medje crossroads, they rounded a bend and Nebobongo came into sight.

The station was to the left of the road, spread over a fairly steep hill. Near the road Winnie could see well planned flower beds and lawns, and beyond were five brick houses. The one on the left, it was explained to her, was a dwelling house for missionaries, the one on the right was for the same purpose, and in the centre were the dispensary, maternity theatre and one of the dormitories. As they drove in she saw behind the houses a mud-walled church and more buildings housing the school, some more dormitories, the untainted children's section of the leper work and the carpenter's shop.

Later she was taken for a three-quarters of an hour walk through gardens of manioc, plantains and rice, and was rewarded by seeing the leper village where the buildings, church, school and huts were all built of mud and local materials. The dispensary was the only brick building. There were kilns and drying sheds in the village, where the lepers were making bricks to transform the other buildings into permanent dwellings.

Winnie sensed an air of purpose, efficiency and freedom about the whole place. Even as she arrived the Africans seemed to appear from nowhere; coming in droves they danced, sang and clapped their hands to welcome her. It was wonderful, for she knew that just five years previously the area had been an entangled mass of virgin forest. Here Percy and Edith Moules had laboured, sweated and prayed in order to bring into being what was now a magnificent compound and a thriving work for God.

Winnie's most important job was to reopen the maternity work at Nebobongo, which had closed down when Mrs Moules had left eighteen months previously. This was quite an undertaking, as she was only just beginning to find her feet with the language and was still unused to African ways and work. But determined to overcome these hindrances, she gathered around her the few girls that Mrs Moules had trained and set herself to put them through as speedy and thorough a "refresher" course as possible.

This was where Winnie's capabilities really came to the surface. She showed herself to be a strong disciplinarian and expected hard work; yet she loved her trainees and gave herself wholeheartedly to them. War was declared on dirt, laziness, unpunctuality and irregular attendance. As a result there were tears and some rebellion. In fact one or two girls felt they could not make the grade and ran off home, but came back later to have another try.

Despite rebellion her nurses achieved a standard of efficiency that was acceptable to the State and Red Cross doctors who gave them their final examinations, and some of these women are still amongst the most capable and reliable of the midwives in the mission. Winnie's standard was always "nothing but the best" and in her demand for the highest she showed no deference to colour of skin. On a couple of occasions she rebuked a visiting Belgian doctor for lack of hospital etiquette, and the workmen about the hospital also knew her word of authority, though they sometimes answered back.

Winnie rushed into the Dawns' house one day not knowing whether to be angry or to laugh.

"The cheek of X!" she said. "I could gladly wring his neck. He had the nerve to say, 'Mama Furaha, if you would talk less and live more we'd believe you'!"

In June 1947, almost a year after her arrival in Congo, Winnie wrote to friends at home: "I now have fifteen nurses. We started lessons for them last week. Some of them have got their Preliminary Certificates and are studying for their final one. This is not an easy task, for these girls know little about study. Besides, all the medical terms are in French and the girls know no French, which makes it harder still.

"Often I find they do the big things well, but the little things, which are usually the ones that matter, are not done. This means going over the same ground almost daily and one of the wearying things we find is the constant repetition. But they are very teachable and anxious to learn and, as responsibility is put upon them, they take it in their stride, doing the work well if they are constantly supervised. One of our great needs is patience!

"I have just been looking around the leper houses to see that they are clean. There are the funniest things on the walls serving the purpose of pictures. Hanging in one house was a writing pad cover in blue with the words 'Mighty Writing Pad' and in another a picture cut out of a newspaper was pinned up. I asked who it was of, but of course, nobody knew!"

As time went on and the nurses' training school proved a success, Winnie's excellent system of training reaped its reward. She was able to write home: "You will be pleased to know that all the nurses passed their exams, including the three for the final examination. Their percentages were 100 per cent, 90 per cent and 85 per cent. The two doctors were full of praise, for which we give God the glory. We are now having a month off from school and then we shall start again. The thing that we covet most in these girls is that they are essentially spiritual."

So her medical work continued. Within a short time, the good reputation of the white lady and her hospital became so widely known that an average of thirty births a month took place in the maternity unit. Although her work was not directly leper work, she also arranged special accommodation for leper mothers and delivered their babies. One of Winnie's relatives wrote to her in 1951, asking if she had much contact with the lepers. She answered: "Oh yes, lots. But I used to have much more to do with them, taking charge of the leper camp on occasions when Arthur Scott was away. But now we have an increase in staff, as Florence Stebbing joined us last year, and it is no longer necessary. Up to about six weeks ago I had the leper women's meeting every week."

Indeed the lepers held a special place of affection in Winnie's heart and she sometimes "broke rules" to make them feel loved and wanted. At Wamba on one visit to the station a band of lepers gathered on the lawn to greet their "Mama Furaha". Winnie and Doris Derbyshire came out of the mission house together and Winnie walked over and shook hands with each one, explaining to Doris later, "I can't bear to think there is a difference between them and us, so I shake hands with them. Please don't mention it to anyone."

In addition to her maternity work, Winnie helped with other departments too. There was the daily dispensary work for the compound folk. Local villagers and Christians, who came in from the surrounding district in ever increasing numbers, were another of her interests. Then there were the post-natal and ante-natal clinics, the daily services and preaching in all the departments, and the training school for nurses to absorb her energies.

But she still found time to assist, whenever possible, in the more general work of the compound. She took her turn with the truck, helping to fetch necessities. Usually it was a trip with the African helpers to the weekly markets to buy food, but on one occasion a missionary travelling from Egbita station found Winnie with the Nebobongo pick-up at one of the rivers. Sand was needed for building operations, and as there was no other driver available she had come out with the workmen to help transport the sand. So as not to waste time, she usually took a portable table and her typewriter on these trips. Many friends received letters which had been typed by a river bank or at the edge of a food market!

To save time in the compound itself she rushed around on the bicycle she had brought with her to Congo. She always cycled at top speed, her rosy cheeks and constant smile a familiar sight as she rushed by. The comment invariably made by the African workmen and nurses as she whirled around the station was "Ooooh!" - as only the African can draw it out! "*Ona! anakwenda kama upepo!*" (Look! She goes like the wind!).

Although the work was so demanding Winnie hated to miss any excitement. The incident of the elephant trek is a case in point. Government permission was given to kill an elephant for food for the lepers twice a year. The hunter came one afternoon saying he had killed an elephant and produced the tail as proof. Immediately carriers were found, mostly from the leper camp, and they prepared to set off. Winnie promptly said she would very much like to go along with Will Dawn and Arthur Scott, so the party set off with Winnie the only woman member.

"None of us realized how far we were going to have to walk," says Will Dawn. "Arthur Scott, Winnie and myself and about fifty carriers made up the total. We took the old truck as far as we could possibly get by road. Then off into the forest we walked. For the first three hours everything went well. I was trailing the men, while Arthur was way up with the leaders. Even I began to tire, and I don't know how poor Winnie stood the pace. She seemed to keep up, though she puffed a good bit at times.

"Then we came to the first big stream and a problem presented itself. Winnie felt unable to wade through the water, and begged me to just leave her beside the road to wait for some of the carriers to come out with the first loads. I said I didn't think it wise and offered to carry her over the stream. I'll never know how I did it, as she wasn't a light weight! But we managed it, and kept up with the stragglers of the group of carriers.

"It was midnight before we finally got through the last of four streams and reached the elephant carcass. I think Winnie was more tired than she was willing to admit, and I was almost the same. By firelight the carcass was cut up into pieces and the carriers began the long trek back. But it was 2.30 the following afternoon when we got out of the forest and back to the truck! On the homeward trip out of the forest we made a carrier chair for Winnie, who travelled in style. She admitted, in spite of this, that she never wanted to see another elephant brought in and I assure you I did not blame her!"

Times like this were few and far between for Winnie. Her calling to serve the Africans demanded a very deep sense of committal and her time at Nebobongo was never her own. She bore a tremendous weight of responsibility during her first term of service, as there was no doctor on the station. Frequently she had to make a quick decision which could mean life or death to a patient, and often at night the nurses would call her to assist with an urgent case.

On one occasion the call came to rush a woman to the Red Cross hospital in the pick-up truck. A Caesarean seemed to be the only thing that would save mother and baby. The distance was about nine miles, and Winnie climbed into the truck with the mother while Will Dawn set off at a terrific pace. Suddenly after only three miles, the headlights went out. Frantically Will jammed on the brakes and jumped out to find the trouble. At least five precious minutes were lost while he banged the dashboard and tried to fiddle with the wires. Nothing happened at first, then mysteriously the lights came on again. Will recalls: "As we set off again along the gravel road a frantic banging on the cab window behind me brought me to a halt. Winnie shouted, 'The baby is coming! Turn around and get back to the mission hospital as quickly as possible.' Well, one is not supposed to panic in such circumstances but I reversed that truck at the double in the first possible space and headed back, just making it in time to get the baby sponged and wrapped while the mother was carried back into the hospital." Will adds reminiscently, "With Winnie around there was never a dull moment!"

4

BATTLES, PHYSICAL AND SPIRITUAL

The six years of Winnie's first stay in the Congo were years full of battles. Alongside the physical battle waged in the hospital against sickness and death, were more personal spiritual battles that engaged Winnie and her associates in their missionary work.

After supper in the evenings they would gather in the Dawn's house to discuss and pray over the day's events. A hymn or two would be sung and someone would read and comment on a passage of Scripture before the final prayer session. Will Dawn remembers Winnie's favourite petition was "Lord, may the Holy Spirit work in our midst so that everything may run as on well oiled wheels."

Winnie's personal battles seemed centred around bereavements and disappointments. She was not introspective by nature, nor was she easily depressed, although on one occasion she did confess to Will Dawn that she had never experienced such a period of loneliness in all her life as the one she had just been through.

"We tried to get her to talk about it in order to find out the root of the trouble," says Will, "but she seemed reticent to do so. Such experiences were rare, and it was strange to hear her come out with such a confession. I cannot recall more than twice, in all the years we worked together as a group at Nebobongo, hearing her with such a despondent note in her voice. Her usual mood was one of joy."

The first "blow" came in 1948 when Winnie, who had been only two years in the Congo, received the news of her mother's death. She was heartbroken, confiding to one of the lady missionaries: "Perhaps if I had not come here my mother would not have died." Another missionary remembers that "she was so overcome that she sat crying on the floor of her room for hours. Eventually some of the African leaders came to her and rebuked her lovingly for her behaviour. She immediately pulled herself together." Two things brought her comfort at that time: the assurance that she was doing the will of God and the knowledge that her "dear Mama" had shown evidence of trusting the Saviour.

Another death that shook her deeply was that of her close friend Edith Moules. The news reached Nebobongo in September 1949 and Winnie commented that it was "stunning, though expected". The news was stunning because Edith Moules' indomitable spirit had seemed unquenchable in the face of tremendous odds, and to Winnie particularly, her vision of the leper work in the Congo had been a constant inspiration.

Such was the spirit of this woman that, after the death of her husband Percy in the Congo and her subsequent return home to England in 1944, she had no desire to settle to a happy retirement. In 1947 she revisited the Congo and Nebobongo in particular, and made full arrangements for leaving the leper colony in the hands of Arthur Scott, who had been joined, of course, by Will and Rhodie Dawn and Winnie. Then, in preparation for spreading the work among lepers to other African states, she set off on a tour of the west coast of the continent.

On her return to England from this long journey she had to undergo a major operation, which revealed the presence of cancer. The doctors warned her that this would probably spread and meant she had only about six months to live. She was not daunted by the news and determined to carry on with her "leper crusade", for she felt sure that it had been inspired by God, and that, fantastic as it might seem, it was His plan that recruits should come forward and leper centres be opened in the countries she had visited. Like the founder of the WEC, she determined to be "a graveyard deserter".

In spite of her physical condition Edith Moules set off on another tour, this time eight months' deputation work in the United States. The doctors had seriously advised against the trip, but she had told them that doing something to try to meet the desperate plight of numerous lepers in the world meant more to her than life itself. On the tour she was often in great agony, but insisted on being taken to meetings in a wheel chair. Before the cancer finally laid her low, she had been instrumental in starting leper stations in nine countries, and all in the space of a few months.

At the memorial service held at Nebobongo a challenge to rededication was given by Arthur Scott. Taking the words "I must work the works of Him that sent me," he emphasized the "must" which had been so evident in the life of Edith Moules. Winnie commented: "After the service I prayed that more than ever I might burn out for Him."

Another test was still to come in which she was personally involved. At Nebobongo for treatment for a tropical ulcer was a man called Zamu. He was the outstanding evangelist of his tribe. Suffering from an incurable ulcerous wound on his right foot, he used to hobble on his left foot and on the big toe of his right with the aid of a stick. In order to get pressure on the big toe, his leg was splayed out at a very awkward angle and gave him much pain. Yet he was one of the most active men on the compound.

He had travelled great distances to preach, his most remarkable journey being to the Walumbi tribe some 180 miles away. Zamu had heard that the Walumbi had never heard the gospel and it burdened him. He said God had spoken to him in the night telling him to go. Winnie loved the story of his interview with the missionary, Miss Esme Roupell, before he left.

"What about your foot, Zamu?"

"God is, white lady."

"But the food is quite different; no palm oil, no salt down there."

"But God is, white lady."

"You might starve or be killed."

"God is, white lady."

And the biggest test of all: "What about your wife, Zamu?"

"She will accompany me. God is, white lady."

The first stage of the journey took them through Ibambi, where Zamu had first found faith in Christ, and where he saw C. T. Studd for the last time. When Mr Studd heard the story of God's call to Zamu he gave him a typical farewell. Rolling up his sleeves he showed him his arms.

"See, Zamu, this arm of mine, once very strong, is now weak and the flesh shrunken. I can't go with you. My time is nearly finished amongst you people. I only go on from day to day as God gives me the strength. So don't depend on me; depend on God. He is with you. He won't die, He will keep you. And don't go with shame! Don't be afraid! Be bold and preach the gospel! Don't drag the flag of God in the earth, but set your face like a soldier to overcome!"

Then he asked; "How many of you are going?"

"Just my wife and I."

"Well, if you are true, God will make you a great company one day."

Zamu and his wife saw that prophecy come true. Amongst the Walumbi tribe a mission station was founded at Opienge, with a church, school, medical centre and more churches in the surrounding district. And now, having returned to Nebobongo, he was having treatment from Winnie. His leg troubled him greatly and she did what she could to relieve the pain. Meanwhile he was as active as ever.

In the Autumn of 1952 he returned to the compound from a conference. The next day he told his wife to cook some food quickly, as he was going to one of the leper camps with "Mama Furaha". A neighbour standing nearby advised him: "You returned only last night and must be very tired. If it were I, I certainly would not go." But Zamu insisted and they set off.

Unbeknown to either of them there was a fault in the brake mechanism of the truck. The vehicle suddenly swerved, turned completely round and toppled over on to its side. Winnie mercifully escaped serious injury but Zamu was trapped in the door. He was unconscious at first but when he came to and was asked, in African fashion, what was his news, his answer characteristically was, "Only good news."

He was brought back to Nebobongo in a critical condition, but without a word of complaint. "Then came the beginning of the end," wrote Winnie, "when it was clear to us that God was going to take him. He told us his journey was over and he exhorted a few of us by name, saying that he had fought his fight for Jesus and it was left for us to fight ours. He passed into God's presence as we sang a hymn of praise."

Winnie's personal affection for Zamu went deep. "Dear Zamu! I knew him for a few months only while he was having treatment, and I always thought of him as being just perfect. Indeed it is true that, even though I looked for faults in him, I couldn't find them. He was on fire for Jesus and souls."

The accident affected her intensely. When people came to say how sorry they were, or mentioned it in conversation, she would weep and weep. She kept indoors, avoiding such contacts as much as possible. But again the African Christians felt this situation could not go on. Frank Cripps was in Nebobongo for the funeral and met Malikumba, a bright leper Christian, hobbling along on his stumps with the aid of a stick. Frank asked where he was going for he knew he was unable to travel about much.

"I am going to see 'Mama Furaha'," Malikumba replied. "When we are sorrowing at the time of death 'Mama Furaha' comes to us with God's word. She cheers us and helps us bear the trial. Now she is in need of cheer and I am going with those same words to bring her comfort." In his mutilated hands was his New Testament, with a slip of paper peeping out of the pages here and there where he had looked up suitable verses which he knew would be a help to Winnie. Frank adds, "I know that Winnie was most appreciative of Malikumba's visit and words of comfort." She was not seen to weep over Zamu's death again.

These more private and personal battles were accompanied by the continual spiritual struggle of Winnie's missionary work. Three factors marked her zeal. She loved preaching and was a splendid evangelist. Prayer had priority in her life; and she had a real love for the Africans.

The evangelism carried on through the maternity work brought her great joy. "Last week we had a testimony meeting," she wrote in October 1949. "It was among the 'waiting women' for those who had trusted God for salvation during the week. There were three of them. I was somewhat amused by the way they referred to the conviction which led them to repentance. They say, 'My heart said to me, Why are you so far from God? It is necessary for you to repent and to trust Jesus to wash away your sins.' "

At another date she wrote: "One of the young women whom we had in the maternity hospital died. She had repented and got right with God while she was here with us, and had stepped out saying that she wanted to finish with the world and serve God. Although married to a polygamist, she witnessed a good confession at home for eighteen months before she died. What a lesson in this death; so often we think that young folk will live to be old and can put off the day of service to the Master. Youth goes as well as age."

By the beginning of March 1952 the re-opened maternity centre had been going for over four years. Winnie conceived the idea of contacting the women who had been through the maternity department and inviting them to a meeting. She wrote to the WEC in London: "I though you would be interested to hear of the conference we had for all the women whose babies had been born in our maternity here. The response to our calling them in was wonderful. About six hundred to seven hundred women with their babies turned up last Friday. Women and babies all over the place!

"We had a meeting about 10 am and many of the women took part. Praise God for every woman who knows Christ as her personal Saviour. We had the next meeting at 2 pm. There were so many women that we decided to have an overflow meeting. A few stayed behind to get right with God. What a wonderful opportunity this afforded of getting the African women together to hear the message of Christ's salvation."

But evangelism in and around the compound thrilled her too. Sunday was her great day for getting out amongst the village people. She loved to walk around the nearby villages or cycle farther afield. At other times she would fill the truck with African preachers, drop them at villages en route, and then preach herself at the furthest point before returning to pick up the others.

On these trips it did not take her long to become quite at home with the people. She would shout a happy greeting as she walked into the village, then join the women at whatever they were doing – cooking, gardening, etc. Often she would sit as they sat, her skirt tucked between her legs, much to the surprise of one of her missionary colleagues, who adds, "The women loved her for it."

Of one of these Sunday outings Winnie wrote: "A week last Sunday I was out at a village some distance away. I took with me a native woman who was able to translate my preaching into the tribal language. I take my hat off to some of these Christian women of Congo, for they are wonderful specimens of what Christ can do. This woman is aflame with love for Christ and is reaching the lost.

"We had as our guide a pygmy man, who was very good to me and led us down the forest paths in order to reach the solitary houses and people. The woman was doing her best to win the pygmy for the Lord. I heard her asking him if he wouldn't like to have a wonderful friend such as she had, meaning Jesus. How my heart thrills over our wonderful salvation; but sometimes I feel so helpless in telling of it because I have only one body and tongue. Yet there is so much to do and so many to reach."

In 1953 Bob and Bess Butters from the United States, who were in the Leper and Medical department of the WEC, visited the Congo for six months. They toured the whole of the WEC field, covering thousands of miles, but spent quite some time at Nebobongo. Extracts from their diary throw light on the battles Winnie faced in her work.

"11.6.53. Up early, breakfast, then off with Winnie to the market where she buys plantains. As we stood around watching the weighing of these, we counted six lepers in all stages of the disease . . . We had wee David with us. His mother died when he was born and now his father is to marry a Christian woman. Winnie is keeping the little fellow until the wedding is over. He is a sweet little fellow and very friendly.

"14.6.53. Two little babies are being held in their mothers' arms; the mothers are badly mutilated lepers. What a future for these babies! yet the mothers do not want to give them up. I felt terrible as Winnie talked to them, for these mites are the only happiness and comfort these people have. I'm afraid I would not see beyond my own longing for something to love, if I were in the same place.

"One young mother with a four-week-old baby could only say, '*Nitangoya kwanza*' (I want to wait a while). The father is willing to give up the child but the mother finds it hard, yet the longer they keep these little ones the harder it is to part with them. This babe is contaminated already, so we didn't press the matter.

"18.6.53. At 4 pm Bob, Winnie and I went out to Chief Baonoku's village. This man has sixty wives and over a hundred children. One of his wives had her baby in for treatment (at Nebobongo) and she accepted the Lord. She wanted Winnie to tell her husband, for she is afraid of him. At first Chief Baonoku was not pleased for he said, 'Why didn't she tell me first?'

" 'She has,' Winnie said. 'She has asked me to tell you right away, for it happened just this afternoon.'

" 'She should have asked me first,' he insisted.

"25.6.53. Chief Baonoku has written a note saying not to bring the woman back today, for he is considering her case. He says he wants her to remain to get the gospel, but Winnie knows this is not his desire. He says he will send for her when he wants her back. We went to his village but he was not there. We left word that we would come a week from today and that he should be dressed to have his picture taken.

"2.7.53. Baonoku's village again. There he was all decked out in his finery. You never saw anything like it. After we finished he had his new young wife brought out and she was decked out with much colour and splendour too. On her head was a hat similar to that of the Chief, but it was covered with red parrot feathers. She held his ivory tusk horn which was beautifully carved. She looked as frightened as could be . . .

"We walked away so Winnie could have another 'quiet' chat with him about his wife who was converted at Nebobongo. He is most upset about it, for this has belittled him before all his people. The idea that a wife of his would do such a thing without first asking permission of *him* has touched a very big thing in his life.

"Winnie told him that such affairs of the heart with God are personal matters, but he would not have it . . . Of course, he says he is glad she is walking with God. She needs to for she has been a most deceitful woman, has committed sin with one of his sons, yet he didn't punish her for it! But now this has been the final stroke and he cannot take her back. Winnie said she would pray before leaving him and asked him to remove his hat. He said he wouldn't.

" 'But,' said Winnie, 'when your people come to you they always remove their hats, don't they?'

"But he said he couldn't, for that was one of their secrets.

"Winnie prayed that the Lord would strike his heart and make it soft, convicting him of his hardness. 'Don't pray like that, white lady,' he said.

"We came away, Winnie very burdened for him, but leaving him to meditate on what had been said. As we had stood talking men and children had been all around us.

"6.8.53. In the afternoon we went to Chief Baonoku's village for chickens and eggs. Winnie had taken the wife and baby back but the Chief would not have her, so Winnie had to take her and the child to her parents' village.

"The Chief was angry so Winnie wasn't going to go near him today, but when we stopped the car by the tree where we do the buying a policeman came saying the Chief would like to see us. We went over and found about a hundred of the chief's *capitas* there in a circle before him all dressed in their feathers and bark-cloths. He had called them in to talk to them about getting their villages cleaned up for the Commissioner, who would be coming soon. But he also wanted his people to see that his heart was all right toward the white lady, so had called her over to him. We stood there and listened.

"Winnie said to him, 'My heart is all right towards you, but your heart is not right towards God, and that is what worries me.' The Chief replied, 'Some day I will have you come over and talk to my people and then you will know I have nothing against you.' Well! If you know Winnie you will realize this was no opportunity to be let slip. She just said to him, 'Oh, I'll preach to them right now'.

"Without a further word from the Chief she turned and addressed all the befeathered men sitting in the circle, and the Lord gave her a voice to speak a straight word to them. There were many children about too. What an opportunity! And how we prayed as she spoke.

"The chief seemed touched and thanked Winnie, but she impressed it upon him that God is doing a mighty thing in Africa and he had better get right with God before it was too late. We left, trusting God for this man's salvation. Two more of his wives are at maternity, one young and one old, and we believe for their salvation too. So far they seem fearful of the meetings because of the situation with the one he has turned away."*

---

* Missionaries and national workers kept contact with the Chief for many years after Winnie left Nebobongo for Opienge. Several of his wives were converted. His fate was a grim one, for he was captured by the Simbas in 1964, tortured terribly and killed.

As Bob and Bess were driving home with Winnie from one of the visits to the Chief, she shared another burden with them. She was concerned for a man for whom she had prayed much and to whom she had talked about the gospel constantly. Each time he would say. "When I have drunk all the wine from my wine palms I will turn to God."

Now this man had been brought in for treatment after having been ill for nearly a week. Winnie had not known he was ill and was shaken to find him already unconscious. She did all she could for him, talking to him in the hope of some response, but there was none. She asked his people to leave him at the hospital so that she could treat him and have further contact with him, but while she was busy they took him away.

The next morning Winnie received news that he had died, but she didn't believe it, for she had not heard the death wail. Bess recalls: "Bob, Winnie and I with one of the teachers from Nebobongo decided we would walk over to the village to see for ourselves. It was getting dark, so we took flashlamps and set out.

"We found his hut crowded with people and the man on a bed with his wife stretched out beside him. He had the death rattle very definitely in his throat and it seemed that the people were sitting about waiting to let out the first wail.

"Winnie called to the man and spoke to him, but got no response. She spoke a few words to the crowd and the teacher translated for her. Then she prayed and they all answered with the customary '*No nkombo na Yesu*' (In the name of Jesus).

"We left the hut then, for there was no point in remaining any longer. Winnie was very upset. In the light of the fire in the hut I saw the keen look of disappointment in her face and the tears brimming in her eyes as we turned and walked out. Just as we reached Nebobongo we heard the wail go out. A soul gone into eternity without Christ – because he had put if off."

Another entry from Bess's diary reveals that Winnie's fear from theatre days was not far away and she had to struggle with it still.

"7.7.53. Winnie came and had a cup of coffee with us. While we were chatting a woman came to our window. She was very agitated and said that her son was desperately ill. Jim Grainger took Winnie in the car to the Greek trader's shop where the boy was. His father is a cook in the shop.

"The boy was very sick and they brought him back in the car. He was raving and throwing himself about and Winnie diagnosed meningitis. She felt helpless. She knew the only answer was penicillin injected into the spinal fluid, but she also knew how hard it was to get the needle in sometimes.

" 'Oh, I can't do it,' she said to us. But she went to her room to pray and returned quietened. The first attempt was a success and the needle slid right into place. Winnie returned immediately to the house, dropped on her knees and thanked the Lord for what He had done. Then she went back to the little family and they got down to prayer. The father was weeping so much he couldn't pray. This is a Christian family and there are two more children. We feel they need so much prayer."

"We feel they need so much prayer." This summed up Winnie's own feelings about the Christians in and around Nebobongo. In the spiritual battle she desired more than anything to see revival amongst the Christians, both missionaries and workers.

"How we long for revival!" she wrote home. "In answer to prayer we have seen a few getting right with God. These are mostly professing Christians who live with us on the station. Recently about six or seven came in desperation about their lukewarmness and lack of communion with God. One was exercised about her thoughts. She said, 'I want God to deliver me from my bad thoughts'.

"I was talking to the young men on the station and asking them when they were going to start burning out for God. Some want to go on with Him, but others – not yet.

"Afterwards, when they were talking amongst themselves, I heard that one had said, 'Let us not take this as the voice of the white lady, but let us take it as the voice of God and humble ourselves before Him and get our hearts right.' "

Winnie's prayers for revival were answered. The year after the shock of Zamu's death a spiritual tornado shook the whole station. The revival of 1953 swept through a large area of the Congo, covering thousands of miles and spreading from mission to mission. The Congolese Church was revived and many were brought to Christ.

Words are inadequate to describe the full impact of that spiritual awakening. To many, God and Jesus Christ became real for the first time. The presence of God's Holy Spirit was "felt" in a new way.

It was evident in the conversation and lives of men and women. It was nothing to hear men in the street talking about God with the same ease as they had once discussed the sports results. Workmen, normally lazy, did more work in one day than they had done in a week. Stolen property was returned in such quantities that government officials were overwhelmed by the amount of tools that had been restored.

Churches were packed and people ran to the meetings in order to get a seat. Church workers were given a new power and children found joy in testifying to their new found Saviour. Conviction of sin and the realization of a need for forgiveness led to the joy of being reconciled to God. There was singing to be heard everywhere at all times, even far into the night, for joy was the keynote. Husbands and wives were reconciled and families united in Christian love.

In all this Winnie was in her element. How she rejoiced at God's blessing at Nebobongo! There had been hidden sin among the people living on the compound and now it was brought to light and forgiveness sought. Often she heard a Christian say, "I would not have confessed this thing for anything, not even under the whip of the Chief, but under the terror of God I cannot hold back."

As a result a new tender relationship sprang up between the missionaries and the Congolese Christian workers. There had always been a good spirit but now it was even better. All were on common ground; all were trusting in the same Jesus Christ; all were accepted before God in the merit of the same Saviour and all were working for the same Master.

But the price of peace of heart was sometimes very costly, as Winnie found out. She shared her experience with Frances Linklater.

"It was Sunday. At the morning service the Lord rebuked me for my behaviour towards a Congolese sister. We had not been getting on well and I had been harbouring unkind thoughts towards her. I felt I had to stand up there and then in that meeting and ask that dear sister to forgive me.

"It was terribly humiliating, and a revelation to me that there was still a good deal of self in me. But as I confessed brokenly before the congregation, the Holy Spirit seemed to burst in upon us and people all over the church began to cry out and ask one another for forgiveness. It was a painful and yet precious experience!"

It was Winnie's sixth year at Nebobongo and her first furlough was due. She viewed it with mixed feelings. She longed to see her family and friends and Coedpoeth, but how could she leave Congo and her people at Nebobongo? The revival had awakened the Christians and she could at least leave with the assurance of their new zeal. But the parting would not be easy.

The furlough party consisting of one married couple and three single women arrived at Ibambi head station for a final briefing and the farewell meeting. Bob and Bess Butters wrote in their diary for that day, October 6th 1953:

"Each one gave a word, Winnie speaking from Luke 10:27: 'Thou shalt love the Lord thy God with all thy heart, and with all thy soul, and with all thy strength, and with all thy mind; and thy neighbour as thyself'.

"It was dark when we came out of the church. As they went to the car the Africans came running from all directions and surrounding it. We had a singing jam of blacks and whites.

The folks could hardly keep the tears back as they said goodbye and got into the car. Poor Winnie especially felt it, for she knows these people so well. I can truthfully say I have never heard such singing. How Winnie managed to get that car through that mob I don't know!"

5

FURLOUGH AND THE CONGO AGAIN

Furlough was a busy time for Winnie. Seeing her father and staying for a while in her beloved Coedpoeth, meeting old friends, making new ones and speaking at meetings filled her days. She also took advantage of a visit to Switzerland for further French study. A friend who met her there commented, "Just the same Winnie but very much more mature."

It was not surprising. Over six years in the mission field had certainly wrought in her a new maturity. Everywhere she went people testified to blessing received through her life and ministry.

After the WEC conference at Glenada, Northern Ireland, a friend wrote: "I first met Winnie at the Glenada conference in 1954 and for me it meant a complete spiritual upheaval." Mr John Lewis, senior, of the WEC saw her and commented: "It was on the stairs of number 32 that we met and the subject of our discussion was precious souls outside the Kingdom not being reached. As we talked Winnie wept. She certainly had the gift of tears for perishing souls and I had not. Her tears I have never forgotten, but since then the Lord has given me tears for souls too."

Her prayerfulness impressed those who knew her on furlough. "Her prayer life was outstanding," wrote one colleague. "I had never seen anything equal to it. She spent hours in prayer while we were together on a tour. I went to her room one morning and receiving no reply to my knock quietly opened the door. There was Winnie prostrate on the floor praying with the hearth rug wrapped around her, for it was a very cold, wet morning."

Pat Holdaway also remembers her habit of prayer. Pat, who was preparing to go to the Congo, was asked to accompany Winnie on a tour of meetings around South Wales. "I was impressed by the amount of time she spent alone with the Lord. We were in Swansea during the cold of winter. I can still see Winnie, sitting indoors with her overcoat on, while having her prayer and meditation time. She allowed nothing to hinder her from it."

Winnie's faith was simple and childlike. She took God at His word and expected Him to respond to her faith. Jock Purves, of the London headquarters, remembers a typical instance. "At the HQ Winnie came to my room one day saying that she was not feeling well. She asked me to anoint her with oil and pray for her healing in the name of the Lord. It seemed an unusual time and place for doing this and I smilingly said so. In her happy way Winnie replied that she did not agree, as that was how she did it in the Congo. Quite informally and naturally, in her medical work, she would anoint mothers and babies in His name, laying hands on them and praying for their healing. I understood her request then and she was anointed and prayed for."

There was still nothing sanctimonious about Winnie. She was always ready to appreciate a funny situation or put embarrassed folks at ease. One such occasion was a meeting for young people in Tongwynlais, South Wales, on a Saturday morning. It proved to be at an inconvenient time, for only three small girls turned up and the meeting threatened to be a flop. The girls were shy and sat mutely looking at each other until the youngest said, "Our cat has got kittens."

The older girl turned to her. "You mustn't talk about that here. This lady is a missionary!" Winnie burst out laughing, treating it as a great joke, and the ice was broken.

Her down-to-earth practicality was as much in evidence at home as in the Congo. Visiting some fellow missionaries at Gowerton she found their baby had a disturbing and stubborn cough. Promptly she took charge of the medical needs, diagnosing the trouble and prescribing a remedy. Her forthrightness was always appreciated even if it was sometimes brusque. For instance, one of her friends at Coedpoeth asked her, "Aren't you afraid of the lepers and leprosy?"

"Afraid?" Winnie said in an astounded voice. "I love every one of them." The friend comments, "She made me feel that high," showing the tip of one small finger.

Indeed Winnie's love of the Congolese was intense and deep. The work she had left behind was constantly in her mind and prayers, and towards the end of the furlough she began to seek the Lord's sanction for her return to Congo. From Coedpoeth she wrote to relatives: "It was last October, when I was being renewed physically, that God gave me the word to 'go quickly, and tell'. As I looked upon the field with a little fear in my heart for all that it might hold, the Lord continued to speak to me from Matthew 28: 'and, behold, He goeth before you.' And then when the disciples got there, the Lord met them and said, 'Be not afraid!'

"Again, as I was praying that the Lord would give guidance concerning the compound to which I should be allocated, I read in the next chapter (Mark 1), 'Behold, I send my messenger before thy face, which shall prepare thy way before thee.' So as you can see, God is going with me and He is also going before me. So I have nothing to fear, have I? Praise His blessed name."

March 1955 saw Winnie setting out on her return trip to the Congo. In the same party were Mr and Mrs Vernon Willson, veteran Congo missionaries, and Elsie Sextone, who was on her first journey to the field. Their journey took them through the Mediterranean Sea and the Red Sea to Mombasa on the east coast of Africa.

Almost three weeks on board ship gave them time to get to know one another. Winnie proved a good companion with her ready chatter and friendliness and Elsie was impressed with her spiritual stature. "As far as I could perceive hers was a consistent walk with the Lord. She knew an intimate contact in prayer with the Lord and her one desire was to make Him known. She would pour out her heart in prayer for the Congolese, whom she loved, often praying aloud in the cabin.

"She was bold and unafraid of what others thought, and spoke freely. During the trip from Nairobi to Mombasa by train, we shared a compartment with an elderly lady who was *not* in sympathy with missionary work. At each stop, and these were very frequent, Winnie would alight and gather a crowd of Africans around her and tell as much as she could of her Saviour's love. She was so loud and spontaneous in the Swahili language that all nearby could hear. And how they listened!

"I was ignorant of the language so could not join in. Instead I prayed in the compartment, rejoicing that I was thus witnessing with her to the people to whom we had been sent. Our travel companion was irate and turned to me in no uncertain manner at each stop, heaping abuse in English upon my head!

"However, this lady was taken sick later in the journey and we both sought to care for her. As we did, her whole attitude changed. She seemed to realize that it must be true that we had God's power within us, or why should we be kind to one who had been objectionable to us?"

Winnie's own comments on the journey, on arrival at Ibambi, were: "I had an uneventful journey through Africa, travelling about a thousand miles or so from the coast through Kenya and Uganda, taking about ten days to accomplish it. You can imagine how slowly we move here.

"We passed through Nebobongo on our way to Ibambi, and how great was our joy in reuniting with our beloved brothers and sisters in Christ there. We hugged each other and we laughed and we cried and we sang for joy, praising our blessed God who had brought us together again after the months of separation." It had been, in fact, over a year since they had last met.

Now came the final decision on her future work. Just before leaving Nebobongo for furlough Winnie had expressed several times her desire to go to work "down south", for Nebobongo was well staffed. Dr Helen Roseveare had arrived at Ibambi and nurses were preparing to come out from the homeland. Winnie was more concerned about places in the south where there was no established medical work. She had prayed earnestly that the decision of the Field Director and his committee concerning her allocation might be the right one. So it was with great joy that she accepted their suggestion that she move 260 miles south to the station at Opienge. That she should be chosen for this station of the four in the south was a special thrill, for this was the area that her friend Zamu and his wife had opened up to the gospel many years previously.

Having said a painful goodbye to her dear friends at Nebobongo, Winnie set out on the long journey in a four-ton truck. driven by a fellow missionary. The first road from Ibambi to Bafwasende was good, as Congo roads went! It had a hard surface of laterite stones, which was grand in the dry season apart from the bowling clouds of red dust whirling behind each vehicle. The dust completely obliterated their vision and Winnie soon discovered that it got into everything, turning passengers into "redskins" before long! In the months ahead she was to find that in the rainy season this surface became very treacherous. Just one tropical storm would cut gullies right across the road in the most unexpected places and compel the driver to pull up sharply, causing the load to lurch and giving passengers the feeling that they were on a storm-bound ship in the Bay of Biscay! She learnt that drivers of heavy vehicles on this road always carried a spare set of springs, for rarely would a trip be completed without at least one leaf spring broken, and that usually the main spring.

But worse was in store. When the truck turned off the main road at Kilometre 229 and took the road in the direction of Opienge, the state of the "highway" deteriorated suddenly. This road, originally excavated by the Belgians to reach the Angumu gold mines some fifty miles beyond Opienge, had nearly seventy-two "bridges" in the seventy mile stretch to Opienge alone. Calling some of these "bridges" is being ultra-generous! Felled trees rolled into position and sometimes covered with planks served to keep vehicles out of the mud or water below. Harry Jones, a missionary who visited Opienge three years later in 1958, comments: "I shall not forget the road from Km 229. At best, when dry, it is a series of hairpin bends. At worst, when wet, it is a nightmare of mud and ruts. Small wonder the rule of the road is one way traffic up or down on alternate days!"

Though about forty of the "bridges" were eventually improved, the Angumu mines were abandoned after Independence in the Congo and the road was unkept, becoming almost impassable. It is still considered one of the worst roads in the WEC area of the Congo. And Winnie was to be linked by this road with those she knew best in the north.

Despite the poor road Winnie was delighted with the changing scenery as the truck bumped its way towards Opienge. The forest through which the road wound was dense and impenetrable, with majestic trees and beautiful evergreen foliage that amazed her. And at the edge of the forest on the roadside stood delicate ferns some ten feet high. Then a colony of baboon appeared on the road ahead, making the most of the open space away from the constant shade of the jungle. They watched the truck approaching, then skipped off into the forest, reappearing on the road after the truck had passed. She caught glimpses of elephants and buffaloes and strained her eyes to see the okapi for which that area of the Congo was world famous. Villages dotted along the road reminded her of the new responsibilities ahead and she waited eagerly for the first view of Opienge.

Eventually Opienge *poste* came into sight. First they saw some small shops and a rice factory owned by Greek traders. A little further along they passed the Belgian administrative offices and flagpole, then the Belgian rest house with its lawns and the open space swept daily by prisoners. On the opposite side of the road Winnie was shown the state dispensary manned by an African male nurse. Half a mile along the road they came, at last, to the mission compound, stretching back at right angles to the road down a fairly deep valley and continuing up the hill on the other side, until it seemed to merge with the forest.

On the flat ground near the road Winnie could see the missionaries' houses, the church, and the other buildings making up the girls' school compound, the dispensary, workmen's village and outhouses; the schoolboys' compound was beyond on the other side of the valley. Most of the buildings were built of brick and all were covered with leaf roofs.

But most of all Winnie was struck by the clean appearance of the station. At Wamba and Nebobongo the soil was a deep, dusty red and a dropped handkerchief was stained and dirty immediately. Here the soil was almost white and of a sandy composition, sparkling in the sun and dazzling her.

Awaiting her arrival were Aubrey and Hulda Brown with their son Ronnie and twins, Ken and Carol. Winnie was warmly welcomed and made to feel at home very quickly. "Auntie Winnie", as she was soon known to the family, settled happily into the work and routine of the compound.

Shut off as they were from the outside world, the "family" organized life to a pattern of work and recreation, giving as much time as possible to the work of the station but also planning fun for the children. Winnie's old love of picnics was soon re-awakened when a picnic to the beautiful Opienge waterfall was arranged.

She was, as always, at the centre of anything new that was happening. When European foodstuffs were a bit short "Auntie Winnie" never failed to concoct something, turning out wonderful cakes and cookies. Her skill in cooking (learnt many years ago from Mama) became well known and her gift for producing something out of nothing was appreciated most of all.

The Browns have precious memories of the time that Winnie was with them. Hulda says, "Winnie helped me bring up my children! At one time the three eldest all had whooping cough badly. I do not know what I would have done without Winnie's care and the injections she gave them. There was a close bond between her and the children and they were always exchanging presents. For one birthday she gave the twins a Swahili New Testament each. Carol's New Testament escaped the hands of the Simba rebels and she has it still, proud that it was dedicated to her in Winnie's own handwriting."

Although Winnie liked to plough her own furrow she loved company. She was perfectly happy at Opienge, where she had full liberty to work out her own plans independently yet return to the family atmosphere of the Browns' home for fellowship. Each evening she would go along there for prayers, except on the night she reserved for letter writing. On Friday evenings the African leaders would join the gathering at the Browns to talk over work, read the Bible and have prayer together. Only medical calls kept Winnie away, and probably these times were the highlight of the week. Sunday evenings were also special, for with the children they would enjoy singing around the little organ.

The Browns recall that "Winnie always had a song. Her name 'Mother Joy' suited her. From our house we could sometimes hear her singing in her own house – it could be early in the morning while brushing her hair – just praising the Lord at the top of her voice. On one of our trips home from Stanleyville she sang most of the two hundred miles! She alternated Swahili and English verses of '*Ninataka kuikala serikani kweli*', a paraphrase of 'Onward Christian Soldiers'."

In quieter mood, Winnie's spiritual life was evident. "She would get up fairly early in the morning so as to have a quiet time of prayer and Bible study and be ready for the first meeting which began at 6.30 am. Again in the evening she would spend a long time in prayer and reading. That was her regular habit, sometimes disrupted in the morning if a medical case had given her a broken night (though gradually she built up an African staff to take care of night calls and she was only disturbed for emergencies). Many times during the day we found her sitting in her living room quietly meditating with her Bible open.

"For a time we used to gather for prayer in the church at 10 am, just the three of us away from station people, door-callers and children. Those were times of intercession for the work and a source of spiritual strength for ourselves. It was also a time when we could talk freely to each other in the presence of the Lord.

"We did not always agree with Winnie on everything; her ways and ours sometimes diverged. She was an individualist and did not like interference in her way of working. On occasion there were demonstrations of self-will and in church meetings she could put a case so strongly that she caused embarrassment.

"She could also 'fly off the handle' when the Africans crossed her. There were times after an outburst when the women would come to ask me to approach Winnie for them, as they were afraid of her severity. But she was so Christ-conscious that differences and problems faded easily. She forgave quickly and wholeheartedly and we never had a difference that was not immediately dealt with.

"The Africans also found this. One of the Opienge evangelists had crossed her and she felt it right to rebuke him. But in doing so she really 'told him off'. Later when she had thought things over she realized she had gone too far. She called the evangelist over and said: 'Samuel, my peace of heart is worth more than whether you or I are right in this matter. I am sorry I spoke to you in the manner I did.' And she asked him to forgive her."

Winnie comments on her new home and work in 1957: "This is a new work for me in a new district – we are just on the equator about 260 miles or more from Nebobongo – and I am doing medical work and girls' school work. Please pray for me as I take up this work that in all things God may be magnified.

"The folks come here in droves for medical help. There has been a small medical work going on here for years, but we are now going to develop it a little and are about to start building a small maternity unit and a small dispensary."

The school work introduced her to a wider responsibility than just teaching. The seventy girls were boarders, so night and day care was necessary. She comments: "I have not done this work before . . . in many ways it will be a case of learning with them!" Winnie employed local Christian women to help with the domestic duties of the school and to be "mothers" to the girls. They supervised them during the days and slept in their dormitories at night but Winnie became their "Big Mother" and personal friend.

But the medical work drew from her new depths of dedication as she planned and budgeted for bigger and better facilities for her patients.

Hulda Brown remembers: "Aubrey and I normally had breakfast around 8 am and from where we sat we could see Winnie at work in the dispensary. Beginning with the preaching service for the patients, this would take her about two hours."

People came to the medical centre from as far as sixty miles away, and Winnie's skill with children's diseases was put to good use. A small building some 150 yards from her own house accommodated her hospitalized patients, but this soon became too small. She obtained plans for a modern maternity block from an architect friend at home, and Aubrey Brown took charge of the building operations. Before the Browns left for furlough in 1959 the building was completed except for the doors and windows. Hulda adds: "Winnie poured her money into this building, determined to make it the best possible . . . One day we talked about tithing with her and learned that she gave to the Lord much more than a tenth of her money. She systematically gave a fifth and then began to give more. It seemed impossible to out-give her, she was so generous."

With the maternity work, a dispensary for about two hundred patients, nurses to train, and post-natal and ante-natal clinics, she was kept even busier than at Nebobongo. "Life is really hectic!" she wrote. "Today being Saturday I have just come away from my three weekly clinics: dispensary, child welfare and ante-natal; so it is a full morning. Last night we had a premature baby. I don't know how it will go on. At the moment it is drinking off a spoon but whether it will continue to do so remains to be seen."

Very often it was these unexpected cases that took up her time. People knew where to ask for help and they would come and stand on her doorstep. If Winnie did not attend to them they would cough as if to say, "There's someone here waiting." Sometimes the sick were carried into the station on improvised stretchers, but once Winnie had her own car this was used to bring patients in quite often. Occasionally she would take an emergency case to Bafwasende, where a doctor was sometimes in residence. The ninety mile drive along the dreadful road was terrifying, especially at night. She usually took a male nurse with her, but it was still an ordeal.

Aubrey remembers one emergency on the compound itself. It was common to have very severe lightning storms in the district and on one such occasion the lightning struck the compound, knocking down five schoolboys. "Winnie was first on the scene, bounding across the quad. When I arrived she was giving artificial respiration to the boys and I helped. There was turmoil around us and wailing, as one young lad was dead. The other four all revived but needed hospital treatment. François owes his life to Winnie. He was severely burned by the lightning, but Winnie made successful skin grafts and treated him for months. As he recovered she taught him tailoring and he became her tailor for the needs of her work."

At times she was brought cases that were beyond human help: "Recently in the night a young lad of fifteen was brought to me. To all appearances he was dying and I laid hands on him and anointed him in the name of the Lord. God wonderfully answered prayer and started to raise him up from that moment.

"Also a woman came in with her baby from a village about sixty miles away; she had managed to get a lift on a lorry. The baby was critically ill with pneumonia. I prayed for it and God answered, so I told her to come in the next day so that we might give thanks to God. Then I spoke to her about her own soul.

She was one who went to church but had never repented. She said that she was ready to repent and forsake her sin, so we prayed together and she was saved."

In all her work Winnie's deepest longing was to see spiritual fruit. Talking of her favourite department, maternity, she would often tell the Browns: "Another woman has gone home today with a beautiful new baby – and a new heart." Hulda continues: "She never lost an opportunity to witness for the Lord. We were out with her in the car one day, and had to stop because of a fallen tree across the road. We all got out and while Aubrey was attending to the removal of the tree Winnie was busy talking to the people nearby about their need of a saviour."

In May 1957 Winnie wrote: "My heart is as a fire. I just long for the salvation of souls. It is my daily cry. Because of my medical and school work, I am not able to get away from the station as often as I would like." She would however walk or cycle into the nearest villages with one or two Christians, when she could find the time. In the villages they would hold an open air service. Winnie was a popular speaker with her happy face, racy speech and evident concern for people's well-being. Sunday was invariably a day for evangelizing and she wrote often about her experiences.

"Last Sunday evening in a village about two kilometres away we had an open air meeting with much freedom. A woman had been saved in that same village in the morning. We sang almost all the way there and then all the way back. We sang up hills and down dales and still didn't seem to be hoarse!"

But it was not always easy to visit the villages. The Walumbi people, relatives of the Mangbetu, were great fighters and at the least provocation knives would appear. One evening Hulda and Winnie had barely started a meeting in one village when a drunken quarrel broke out. "While Hulda was getting on with the meeting I was occupied in separating the fighters and drawing the leader out of the village by the hand," says Winnie, adding: "Missionary life is not all sunshine. In fact we have a terrific amount of cloud."

Many missionaries had worked at Opienge before Winnie, and she was quick to appreciate this. "The word has been faithfully preached in this area for the past twenty years, and so the people are ready to believe if we will go and find them and persuade them. Because of this my heart is just brimming over with gratitude to God . . ." Then she goes on to write of various people who have recently found salvation. "One of these was a terrible harlot, known far and wide for her bad life . . . another is a policeman who was guarding the prisoners. Apparently he had been in the conference meetings held in his village last week and put up his hand to indicate that he wanted to repent, but someone had pulled it down saying, 'Don't repent.' But God got His man. He got him tonight. And he told us his story, saying that the people used to call him Satan because of his terrible fighting and because he was a policeman. As he had a measure of authority over the people you can imagine how he would vent his hatred on them. He said people hated him because he was such a blackguard. He confessed that he was also a terrible drunkard.

"Please, oh please, I do ask you to pray for these people. Lots and lots of them have come to the Lord during these last months, almost all of them through personal contact, sometimes as many as three a day. Most of them are patients or relatives of patients."

Winnie's concern was people. She felt and prayed for each one she treated, grieving and rejoicing with them. A missionary on a visit to the station found her weeping over a woman in the maternity unit who had lost her baby. Winnie had done all she could to no avail, but it was more than just another case to her. An incident that upset her terribly was the tragic death of the "bright, intelligent and sturdy child of a Christian couple living just off our station.

"He was eating some plantain and rubbing the grease on his mother's Bible (he was just under two). His mother rebuked him and he started to cry, coughed violently and died just as quickly as that. Apparently the food got into his wind pipe and he suffocated. They ran to me with him but he was already gone. The parents, as you can guess, are stricken with grief; they loved the baby, especially the father who is passionately fond of children."

Winnie rejoiced when those she had prayed for found joy in faith. "Last week I was in touch with a policeman who repented when I first came down here to Opienge, but had fallen away.

"From conversation with him I saw he was spiritually hungry, or apparently so, and I suggested that he should come to get right with God on Sunday. He was there on Sunday for the three meetings and at the 2 pm meeting he got up to testify, asking the Lord to forgive him. This was thrilling to me."

As at Nebobongo, witchcraft and false cults made these victories seem more precious. "One evening one of the workers and I went around a roadmen's village which is just above our station. Three people repented that night and there was joy in heaven and in our hearts also.

"One of the men, whose name is Malobani, was a dreadfully heavy drinker and no matter what he did he hadn't been able to stop. The other day when I asked him how he was getting on and if he still had victory over drink he replied joyfully that he had. 'When I was unsaved,' he said, 'I once swore by witchcraft that I would never again touch drink. But it was no good. I could not resist it. Now God has completely delivered me.'

"Malobani went on to tell me how the lorry driver who takes them to work tried to make him drink by offering him wine and pressing him to take it.

"Malobani just walked way. The lorry driver laughed and said 'So it's like that, is it?'

"'Yes, it's like that', Malobani said with a smile."

Kitawala was a name to strike fear into many Congolese living in the area. It was a cult of witchcraft with extremely vile practices, endless taboos and much secrecy. It was the cause of a lot of persecution of Christians and also became anti-government. Periodically soldiers were sent to round up the members of the cult and place them in concentration camps. These camps were grim places, with drink, women, witchcraft and fighting causing endless trouble.

Winnie was as concerned for the *Kitawala* folks as she was for the other local people, and she was to see transformations in the lives of some of those she spoke to in camp. A man and his wife were converted and Winnie wrote: "The wife, whose name is Maria, had a quarrel with the other women in the camp and the women swore that she would be bitten by a snake that same day. At midday a snake bit her and she was taken to the state dispensary. That night she felt very sick and cried to God to save her and to forgive her sins, saying that she never wanted anything to do with the *Kitawala* folks again.

"When the *Kitawala* folk came to see her she drove them away, and when daylight came she sent for me. I went to see her and prayed with her. Her husband came in from the camp to see her and I spoke to him for some time about his soul. Eventually he said that he would like to repent and that he wanted to come to the mission to take his stand openly.

"I brought him to my house and called a couple of teachers. The man opened his heart to the Lord; then, at the 2 pm meeting (it was a Sunday), he openly testified before the congregation. How our hearts sang for joy, for they are the first ones to repent from the concentration camp."

She wrote about work among prisoners. "I go to the prison every Sunday evening for a meeting. When I went two weeks ago six people responded to the gospel appeal. I had been to another little prison previously and as a result one prisoner was saved and two wives of policemen." So Winnie's love and concern reached out to people not immediately under her care.

The local people in and around the compound knew her practical help as well as her spiritual advice. "Our folk are having great difficulty with their gardens because wild animals come and pluck up their crops. There is one member of the monkey family, a huge beast, bigger than a man, which is constantly in the garden tearing up the plantains, sweet potatoes and manioc. It even digs up the peanuts before they are ripe."

To help catch the culprits she gave the children a day off school, and while the girls went fishing the boys went hunting. "Up to the moment the boys have been in with three monkeys which they caught destroying the gardens. Now they have gone after the other party which left at 3.30 this morning to catch the bigger animals with a net." When the parties returned that night with their catch she enjoyed listening to their hilarious stories of the hunt and sharing some of the meat.

Not only was Winnie concerned with the Africans at Opienge; she cared equally for the white people she met at the *poste.* There were a few Belgian officials and planters and also some Greeks, who had small shops, stores and a rice factory. Winnie became a great favourite and one of the Belgians named his daughter after her.

In her letters she mentions "a young Belgian Roman Catholic, a good man and religious, but completely in the dark concerning things spiritual. How my heart goes out to him, for the poor fellow says it is so difficult, almost impossible, to please God on this earth.

"He says, 'As soon as I put my foot on the first rung of the ladder to climb up to God – I fall down again. I think one must go into a monastery to live a life pleasing to God.'

"I pointed out to him from Scripture that he needed to be 'born again'. He had never heard of it, yet I really believe that he yearns to please God. He had just no idea of the Bible's wonderful writings and says it is impossible to understand anyway without an interpreter."

Amid the varying demands made on her faith Winnie found the local Christians were a constant encouragement to her. Most of them had taken a stand for Christ at much cost. Their zeal was revealed in unexpected ways and she marvelled at their hunger for spiritual food. A week of concentrated Bible study was being held at Nala, three hundred miles away, and invitations were sent around the mission stations to the Christian workers. The Opienge workers wanted to go but there was no transport available. Overcoming their disappointment, they set out to walk the whole way with their bundles on their shoulders. The bundles contained their shoes, which they feared would wear out on the long journey! They covered the distance in about ten days, and what a welcome they received from the Christians from many tribes gathered at Nala! It was small wonder that the conference was a success. They had the luxury of a ride home and Winnie wrote, "They returned full of the fire and zeal of the Holy Ghost and brimming over with joy."

The need for transport was always a problem and Winnie was glad when she succeeded in buying a car. It was an Opel Caravan and had one great disadvantage. It was very low built and had to be driven with great care on the bad roads. But still it enabled her to get about and take a holiday. With another missionary she visited the beautiful Kivu Province to the south of Opienge. "The holiday has done me good," she wrote. "We have travelled about 1,200 kilometres or more. Sometimes we were high up on the tops of the mountains and travelling through cloud. Because the cloud was low and it was raining we could only move at about ten miles per hour. One side of the road was a precipice, on the other side was solid rock and underfoot, slippery sludge! Quite a journey I can tell you.

"Last Monday we went to the Albert Park Reserve to see the animals. We had to stop on the road to wait for an elephant to move off and saw lots of other elephants on the roadside. Hippopotami, too, were just on the roadside and we saw water buck, water hogs, and any amount of deer and buffalo. It was quite enjoyable. Our boys who came with us were very excited, and so amazed at the tameness of the animals. They were also surprised that there were so many animals and nobody killing them. They are used to killing animals from the moment they are sighted."

6

EVACUATION

"The situation here is often tense these days; one wonders what will come next . . . You may have heard of the riots in Stanleyville. It is all because of the desire for independence. My fellow missionaries here in Opienge are leaving for furlough in about two weeks." Winnie wrote these words at the end of 1959 as important political changes were taking place in the Congo.

Hulda Brown recalls: "As soon as we knew we were to leave for furlough in December 1959, we called Winnie and told her. Things were already getting difficult in our area prior to Independence 1960 . . . I remember she put her head on the table for a while, for she knew what this meant for her. We felt badly too, but knew we should get out of there with our four children."

Realizing Winnie's need of assurance, Aubrey Brown called Pastor Alieni Paul in. "We have to leave Opienge now and the white lady will have to stay on her own. Will you take care of her?"

"*Bwana*, we have *mikuki* (spears) too!" Alieni replied. It was a Walumbi way of saying, "You can safely leave her with us. We shall look after her." In fact he was almost offended that they had thought he would not look after her, and proved a man of his word in the years ahead.

The little group of missionaries had been unable to follow all the changes that were taking place. Shut away on their bush station, occupied with their mission of love and service, they asked for nothing more than to be allowed to live and give themselves for the betterment of the people around. And the people were happy to have them.

Apart from radio broadcasts from Radio Stanleyville and Radio Brazzaville (which were often confusing), and occasional visits to or from the white people at the *poste*, they were cut off. All they heard was the far distant rumblings of the possible approach of a storm. Names such as Lumumba, Kasavubu, Gizenge, Adoula, Gbenye or Tshombe meant very little to them. But great social, economic and political changes had been and were still occurring throughout the country.

A set of major events had set a revolution in motion. In 1958 the Congolese had awoken to new possibilities and begun to form their own political parties. In a speech at Brazzaville on August 28th 1958, General de Gaulle had offered independence to any of the French colonies that wished it. As Brazzaville is just the other side of the Congo River from Leopoldville (Kinshasa), the Congolese leaders could not but be affected by this gesture. In that summer many of the Congolese *évolués* had been invited to attend the Brussels Exhibition. The contacts made then moulded the thinking and politics of many.

Then came the Pan African Conference at Accra when "Africa for the Africans" was the slogan. Patrice Lumumba, leader of the *Mouvenent National Congolais*, was present. He was a brilliant orator and returned to the Congo to inflame the population with his fiery speeches.

On January 4th 1959 riots broke out in Leopoldville. Delinquent, unemployed, hungry youths (precursors of the *Jeunesse* groups which were to spring up all over the country) ran through the streets shouting "*Uhuru*!" (Freedom!) They plundered shops, set fire to hospitals, schools and churches, killing many people of different nationalities and creating anarchy.

Their Swahili word "*uhuru*" meant for them freedom from the whites, from hunger and from work. It was in this sense that they interpreted independence. Their conception had a Utopian touch of magic about it. They would have plenty of money for no work, and also white men's cars, shops, villas and even their wives. In scores of cases deposits were made by gullible Congolese to guarantee that certain objects and white women would be theirs after the wonderful day of independence.

More riots broke out in Stanleyville and other places in October 1959. A wave of terror spread through Leopoldville as well and European women and children began to move out of the country. In an attempt to pull things together the Belgian Government called a round table conference in Brussels. This took place in January and February 1960. Forty-five delegates were present, including fourteen Congolese political party representatives and chiefs from the six provinces. At this conference the Belgians' previous suggestion of independence in thirty years, then amended hastily to five years, faded completely before the demand for immediate independence. In an explosive atmosphere and under almost inescapable pressure the Belgians agreed to grant independence in six months' time, June 1960.

From that time until June 30th, Independence Day, the country was caught up in the full force of the political hurricane which ushered in the new era with Patrice Lumumba as Prime Minister and Joseph Kasavubu as President.

In the Orientale Province where Opienge and Nebobongo were situated, Lumumba's agents set themselves up in all the important towns and *postes*. They visited factories and shops enquiring of employees how they were being treated by their employers. Then they drew up lists of those who would be dealt with on and after Independence Day.

They came to the mission stations, interviewed the missionaries, then left to tour the town with public address system blaring, "X is undesirable . . . his name is on the black list." The feeling of insecurity grew, not only amongst the Europeans but also among the better class Congolese. Rumours were numerous and so wild that no one knew just what was happening. Rowdy groups of *Jeunesse MNC* came into the mission houses without warning or consent. They would sit on any chair of their choice and make themselves disagreeable by carrying on a noisy and insulting harangue against the whites.

Winnie had some of these unpleasant visits from what she called the "brass hats". She was alone now at Opienge, as the Browns had left in December 1959. It was a nerve-racking time and the atmosphere was charged with tension. As a result the field leader, Mr Jack Scholes, wrote to suggest that she move to Bomili station to be with Cliff and Peggy White until the unsettled period of Independence Day was over. Winnie agreed to go for two weeks.

Cliff writes: "We were so glad to have Winnie with us, for there was a strong anti-white feeling among the *Kitawala* folk at Opienge. She stayed with us for a fortnight and I did some repairs to her car, while she helped Florence Stebbing with the medical work. Several times I took her out to the villages for emergencies, accidents and illnesses. Our boys loved her and so did the Babari. Her joy in the Lord was so infectious that the whole station seemed to catch it."

On the eve of Independence Day at the end of June both blacks and whites were gripped by a sinister feeling of suspense. Tomorrow, Independence Day, they could expect anything. But the day came and went quite peacefully with some celebrations, of course, mainly in the cities and towns. The forecasts of violence appeared to be false, although there had been incidents in and around Kinshasa, caused mainly by Lumumba's vitriolic speech in the presence of King Baudouin at the Independence celebration. On the mission stations it had been a happy, festive day with the hoisting of the new flag, athletic sports and side shows. There seemed every possibility that the storm clouds would pass quickly, and Winnie, in the light of this, was allowed to return to Opienge.

Four days later the whole country was thrown into uncontrollable chaos. The *Force Public* (National Army) revolted on the grounds that promises of better conditions had been made to most public servants but not to them. As if by mutual agreement throughout the six provinces the army rose against its white officers. These were arrested and ill-treated, their wives raped, some repeatedly in the presence of terrified children, and then their property was looted. Magazines were broken into and trigger-mad soldiers appeared everywhere with rifles and machine guns. Civilians were held up and robbed in the streets and houses were burgled.

Terror and disruption reigned. In one week between thirty thousand and forty thousand white people fled from the country.

The whites at Opienge *poste* sent a note over to Winnie. "We are getting out now while there is still a chance. Come with us."

Poor Winnie was dazed. What was she to do? Unable to assess the true situation and hearing a hundred wild rumours of what was happening to the white women, she felt utterly confused. She knew that, having been five years in the field, her time for furlough could not be too far away, but was she right to leave her people at this moment?

The answer seemed to come when the Belgian Administrator dashed into the compound and summarily said, "*Mademoiselle, c'est un ordre.* You must leave immediately. You have no time even to pack away your things. We are all going and you must join our convoy."

Winnie was in a whirl. In no time she was in her Opel car, lined up with the Belgians and Greeks and on her way to the nearest airfield at Paulis (Isiro) three hundred miles away. The date was July 13th 1960.

The convoy picked up other cars at Bafwasende and continued on. The Africans who lived in villages along the road had no means of knowing what was happening, and were terrified at seeing the whites fleeing in this manner. The route went by the WEC station at Wamba. At the sign "Mission Protestante HAM" (Heart of Africa Mission, as the WEC is known in Congo), Winnie left the convoy and pulled into the compound. She was astonished to find the missionaries still there and everything in normal working order.

"Don't you know what is happening?" she cried. "You ought to be getting out of here."

The missionaries on the station at the time were Daisy Kingdon, Bill and Doris Derbyshire with baby Brian, Geneva

Hilton, my wife, our son Glyn and myself. We were in close touch with the Belgian officials in the town less than a mile away and on Winnie's arrival I went again to the town to glean fresh news. The Administrator said that the Belgian women and children had left the previous day and the Greek woman and children that same morning, for the troops at Watsa camp had revolted and were moving in our direction. In their wake they were leaving the usual sordid trail. He urged me to get the women and children away.

Back at the compound we held consultation. We decided that Winnie should proceed on to Ibambi head station with a report to the field leader. The next day we all had orders to come at once to Ibambi to talk things over. Missionaries from about five stations met there and the Acting Field Leader, Jim Grainger, put to us the words of Mary at the wedding at Cana, "Whatsoever He saith unto you, do it."

Twenty-seven adults and four children left at 5.30 the following morning for Paulis (Isiro) airfield. The convoy which Winnie had travelled with had already left by plane, their cars sold for a song, cameras exchanged for a handful of bananas. We spent the whole day at the airfield waiting for a promised plane. Towards evening the British Consulate got word through to us that there would be no plane coming that day. At the same time the voice of the American Ambassador came over the radio urging all American citizens to get out of the country. The situation was obviously critical and a quick decision had to be made. It was decided to get into the cars and make a dash for the Uganda border six hundred miles away.

It was 9 pm when the convoy set off, Winnie, Geneva, my wife, Glyn and I travelling in Winnie's car. What a journey! We drove until dawn, when we stopped at a quiet spot, got out a couple of primus stoves and made some tea. Hastening on again, we discussed the possibility of danger from soldiers in a military zone through which we had to pass. Belgians had gone that way before us and had been maltreated, so we wondered what was going to happen to us. We talked, prayed, sang hymns

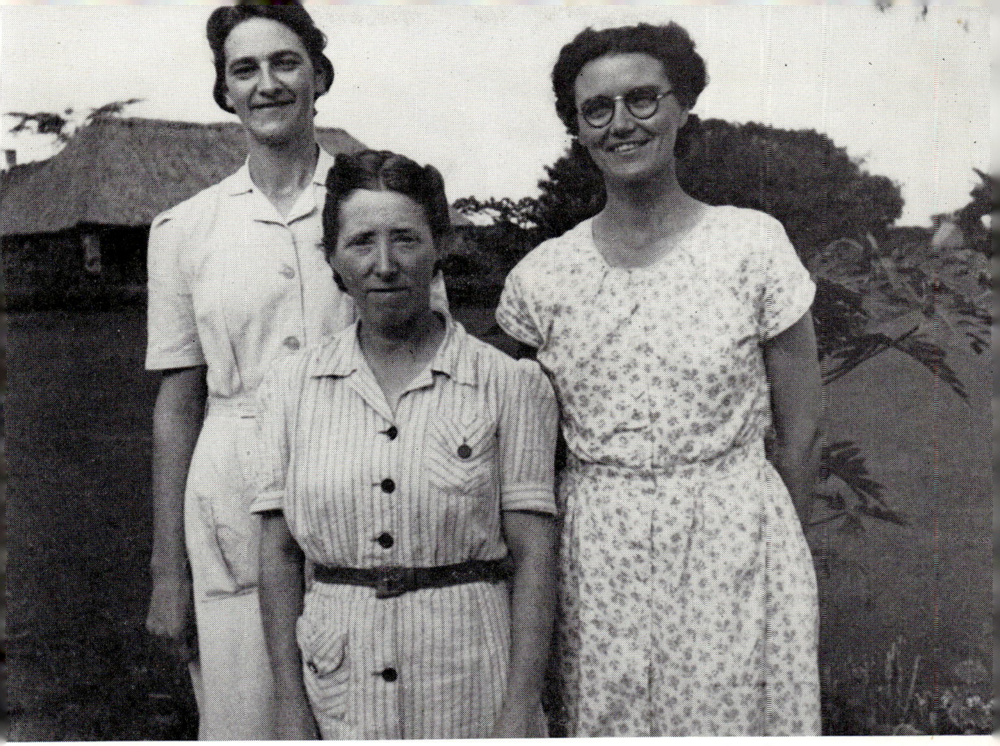

Ida Gibbs (now Mrs Grainger), Florence Stebbing and Winnie Davies, nurse colleagues at Nebobongo medical centre in 1951. One of the missionary dwelling houses is in the background.

Winnie successfully trained only partly educated girls to take the Belgian State examination for nurses. Here are the first five who gained 90 per cent, 85 per cent and 80 per cent.

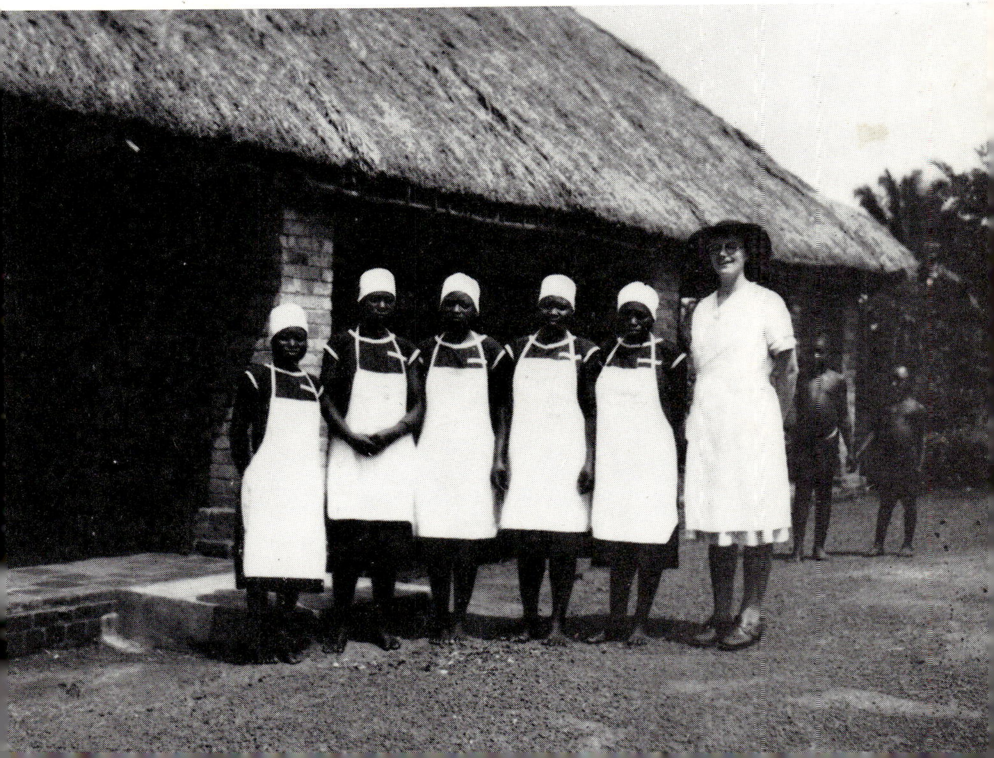

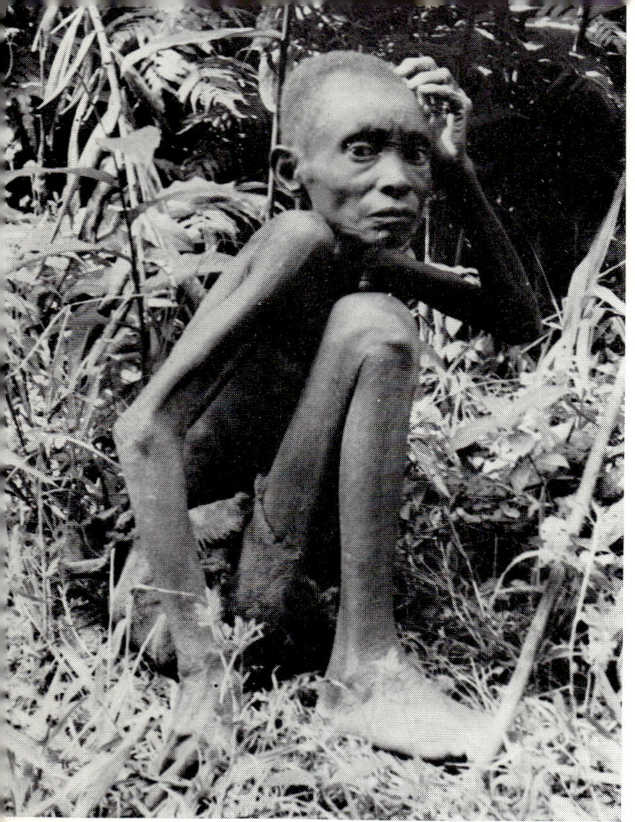

Aftermath of Simba occupation. Thousands of emaciated Congolese emerged after 19 months of hiding in the forest. They survived by eating what they could find. Others died of hunger and exposure.

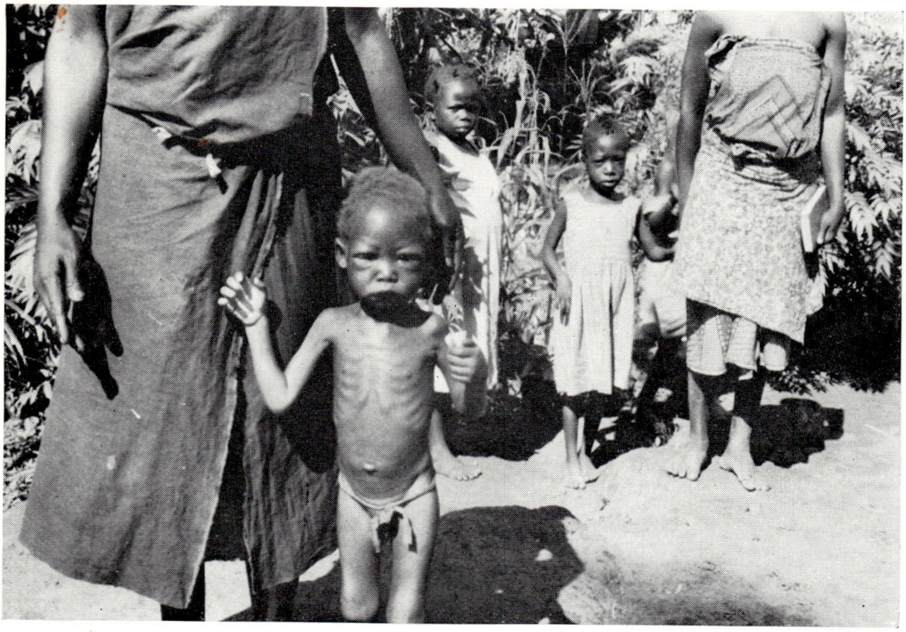

Some of the children rescued after the Simba defeat were thin beyond recognition, suffering from diseases and with their black hair turned white.

and quoted Bible verses for comfort, but the thought recurred, "It happened to the Belgians so why should we expect to escape?" Apprehension began to take over and we again resorted to prayer and encouraging ourselves with hymns and texts. Suddenly we remembered the previous Monday's fellowship meeting at Wamba. We had studied Psalm 34 and verse seven had stood out: "The angel of the Lord encampeth round about them that fear Him, and delivereth them." We sensed that God had given us a promise, and drove along with new hope.

The sun was high and it was hot – as it can only be in the tropics – with a clear bright sky. Without warning a cloud appeared and covered the sun. There was a flash of lightning and a burst of thunder. In a very short time we were caught in a violent tropical storm, and the roads became rushing streams. We continued to drive slowly and carefully, and suddenly we found ourselves in the military camp! There was not a soldier in sight and on we went, through the camp, past the villages and on to the open spaces beyond.

Just as suddenly the rain ceased and the cloud moved away. The sun came out and we were safe. The angel of the Lord had delivered us. The sudden tropical storm after a very hot morning had caused the temperature to drop considerably. The Africans, lightly clad for the heat, feel the cold acutely. When the storm struck the soldiers were huddled in the huts and we escaped their attention.

Might this have been a coincidence? Not with God in control. On at least three occasions while on furlough we were approached by friends who asked, "What was happening to you on July 16th during the morning?" Another said, "I was doing my housework. There was such a burden of prayer for you that I had to leave my work to pray." Suddenly, they said, the need for prayer ceased and the burden on their spirit lifted. By comparing dates and times we discovered that their prayers had coincided with our time of need on that day of flight to Uganda.

The rain storm was not the only sign of God's help that day.

In the afternoon, as we rounded a bend we were suddenly confronted with a huge twelve-wheeled truck sprawled across the road, with a deep ditch on one side and an impassable rise of hill on the other. We still had a hundred miles to go and our spirits sank.

Working as quickly as possible the men felled trees and the women carried stones in an attempt to fill the ditch. This enabled us to get the cars around. We attempted to get a four-ton lorry round but it got stuck and then turned on its side. It was loaded with drums of petrol and the luggage of those of our party who were already prepared for furlough when the evacuation was set in motion.

What were we to do? Leave it all behind or waste more time trying to salvage it?. We realized our first concern was to get the women and children over the border into safety; moreover some local natives had gathered by this time, making it an uncomfortable situation. As there were no soldiers around two of the men volunteered to remain with the lorry while the rest pushed on to the border; they would return to see what could be done with the lorry once the women and children were safe.

Near midnight we crossed over the boundary into friendly territory. The Europeans were wonderful to us, supplying us first with hot cups of tea and meals, then with accommodation for the women in an empty dispensary. There they rolled themselves up in blankets and tried to get some sleep on the concrete floor.

To our joy, a couple of hours after our arrival the four-ton lorry was driven in! A huge truck carrying breakdown tackle just "happened" to come along, pulled the sprawled truck clear and hauled our lorry out of the ditch. We thanked God again for His goodness.

Working among the refugees the Red Cross workers were doing a marvellous job. They clothed and fed us, then arranged accommodation all the way to Kampala and Nairobi. The Europeans opened their homes to us and at one house we were met with: "Oh, what a relief you're English! All our previous refugee visitors were Belgians. We could not speak French and they could not speak English!"

Thousands of refugees – Belgians, Greeks and Portuguese – were still flooding into the country. Shocked groups were everywhere sharing news and experiences. Tragic stories were unfolded. A woman sitting near to us was sobbing quietly to herself. In answer to our enquiry she said in French, "I last saw my husband running in the streets at Stanleyville. I do not know what has happened to him." Little children, tired and hungry, were crying themselves to sleep, not knowing where their parents were. One Belgian told us, "I had a paw-paw and palm tree plantation. I escaped by car when the natives with spears came swarming into the plantation. I stopped the car along the road, looked back and saw my house destroyed by fire." He had lost everything.

Some of our missionaries remained in Uganda in the hope of being able to re-enter Congo when the chaos was under control. The rest of us, including Winnie, flew home to England.

7

STRANGE FURLOUGH

Winnie had been due for furlough, but this second stay at home was not easy to accept. She felt she had been torn from her friends at Opienge, leaving them uncared for medically and spiritually. Her thoughts turned to them continually. There were mothers waiting in the maternity . . . if only there was someone to take over in her absence . . . patients would come to the dispensary . . .

Three days after arriving in London she wrote: "I arrived in England on Wednesday after having driven out of Congo. God was with us and preserved us from all harm and danger. Please will you pray with me that I shall quickly be able to get back to Congo. I am thinking so much about them and their lack of medical treatment and maternity help. My heart is there with them so please pray that God will get me back."

And in a circular letter written the following month: "I would like to get back to Congo as soon as possible. That is, as soon as the situation becomes safe. I don't want this 'furlough' to be a long one. I would like to return even within three months or so."

Winnie's restlessness was fanned by the letters she received from the Congo. "Yesterday I received once again letters from my Congolese friends. They are well, but they do so plead with me to return to them quickly. They tell me that they are waiting for me as children wait for their mother who has gone to work in the garden! They may be more encouraged now, as three missionaries have gone there for the time being and will be helping with the medical work."

The fact that other missionaries had been able to move to Opienge to help during her absence eased her mind a little, but she still took advantage of the WEC staff meeting she attended to press her point.

Jock Purves was present and recalls her intensity and determination. At an opportune moment during the discussions Winnie rose from her seat and said, "Brothers and sisters, I would like you, in your consideration of my case, to wish me God-speed in my return soon to Congo. I have my fare to go and I have already been at home three months, which is far too long. Do wish me God-speed and let me get back as soon as possible."

"Three months! We looked at her in astonishment and admiration but could not agree with her request. The committee said that she needed a longer time at home. Winnie replied that she did not think so and was quite joyfully adamant about it. We eventually agreed that she could go back if she had a letter from the Congolese brethren requesting her return to them."

Winnie left the staff meeting and lost no time in writing to the Congo, determined to place the required letter before Mr Len Moules, the Secretary of the WEC, as soon as possible. But though the letter came, the news which reached Great Britain of the conditions in the Congo was very disturbing. Winnie was troubled over her next step. In January 1961 she wrote: "For the present at least there will be no returning to the Congo. As you know, the situation seems to deteriorate daily. I have therefore put myself at the disposal of the Lord regarding any future service. I have told Him that I am ready to go anywhere He may lead. Indeed a chorus that is often in my heart these days is this (I'm not sure of the order of the words):

> I'll go where you want me to go, dear Lord,
> I'll say what you want me to say.
> I'll do what you want me to do, dear Lord,
> I'll be what you want me to be.

What swayed her mind in particular was the news that some of her colleagues were being maltreated in the Congo and that some missions were redirecting their evacuated missionaries to other countries.

WEC missionaries Mrs Harrison and Muriel Harman were roughly handled, insulted, imprisoned and then put to hard labour with the common prisoners. Frank Bakes was held prisoner on the false charge that his pass was a forgery. The rebels took off his shoes, shirt and hat and made him work at cutting grass and carrying refuse. After this they decided to take him to the town in their car, stopping at every village to show their "catch" and tell the people what a bad man he was. Peggy White at Bomili, where Winnie had stayed, wrote: "The Congolese Administrator and two soldiers came looking for guns. We had none, but we had a Belgian trader staying with us for the night. (He had brought his wife up to see Florence Stebbing.) As soon as one of the soldiers saw him (and giving him no chance to say whether he had a gun or not) he began to torture him. Cliff was helpless to do anything and fortunately the children were in the bedroom and could only hear the shouts of the soldiers. Eventually they left us, saying they would return that night to take him to get his gun at his home.

"After they had left we all had prayer together and waited. Our pastor and one of our evangelists waited with us and four of the young men on the station said they would not go to bed until the soldiers had gone. Florence Stebbing and I stayed with the children, who eventually went to sleep.

"At 2 am we heard the car coming, and the young men came in and stood on each side of our own boys, ready to carry them off out of the house at the first sign of trouble. We saw a miracle that night. The group told the trader he could go the next day to get his gun to hand it in, and the soldier who made all the noise before hardly opened his mouth. Then the Administrator sat down and wrote us out a pass to go anywhere in the Republique du Congo! (He had said previously that we could only have one if we went to Bafwasende to get it.)"

From Nebobongo, Winnie's old station, Dr Helen Roseveare wrote: "Tensions and anxieties, hopes and fears mingle daily as the news changes from hour to hour. If it is difficult at home to follow all the intricacies, it is far harder out here when you are in the midst of them. The situation bristles with difficulties. Economically, chaos reigns; shops are rapidly emptying, prices rising, yet God is still on the Throne!

"The word of today on everyone's lips is *Uhuru*, but with little understanding. Wherever I go, on bike or on foot, anyone I pass in the forest or town shouts out 'Uhuru' and throws his arms in the air. I respond in like manner, we beam at each other and I pass on unmolested."

By June that same year, the news from the Congo was more encouraging and Winnie's hopes of returning rose. Jim Grainger (Acting Field Leader in the Congo) wrote to say that if everything remained quiet for another month he would be giving the "green light" for missionaries to return. Two weeks later Winnie revealed her own feelings on the subject when she wrote: "I had always said that I would have to receive a very definite word from God before I returned to Congo, owing to changing conditions and Church leadership (over which one rejoices). So I got before God in a very definite way, asking Him to clinch the matter regarding my return to Congo.

"On the second day of my waiting upon God He did clinch the matter through Isaiah 48 : 16, 17: 'And now the Lord God, and His Spirit, hath sent me . . . I am the Lord thy God . . . which leadeth thee by the way that thou shouldest go.'

"I knew it was God's voice to me, and so I went to tell the Secretary that I would be ready to return as soon as the way was open for me."

In about a month's time, in July 1961, she was on her way back to the Congo. Her twelve-month furlough had been almost as busy as the first, apart from the first three months when she had taken a complete rest. For the other nine months she had been engaged in tours of meetings, visitation and helping in the work of the Christian Literature Crusade in London.

As she travelled she made new friends and strengthened old friendships. If a person's character can be evaluated by the company she keeps, Winnie's character can be estimated by the friends she made. One of her most valued friends was Briallen

Thomas of Penydarren, Merthyr Tydfil. Very poor by living standards of the day and in constant pain through an uncurable illness, Briallen had made many rich through her sacrifices and selflessness. Limited in the extent of her usefulness by her circumstances, Briallen asked God to enable her to do something for Him. He showed her that she could help by knitting blankets, preparing bandages for leper work, turning old Christmas cards into money and numerous other jobs. Then through a friend Briallen received her great treasure, a budgie which she named Blokie. She taught Blokie to speak and to sing. In Welsh and English Blokie recited hymns and verses of Scripture and spoke with such unusual clarity that he was recorded for the BBC radio and television.

After Briallen and Winnie had met and become firm friends Blokie readily learnt to say Winnie's name and quote various needs: "Winnie needs blankets for the lepers. Winnie needs bandages," or bilingually "*Mae Blokie yn mofyn te i Winnie yn y Congo*! – Blokie wants tea for Winnie in the Congo!" This performance in front of numerous audiences resulted in tea-chests of blankets, bandages and clothes, plus food parcels, being sent out to Winnie and other missionaries.

One Christmas Blokie heard on the radio, "Christmas is coming . . . please put a penny in the old man's hat." With a bit of training the phrase was changed to "Please put a penny in the box!" He would hop on to the missionary box and repeat this refrain and few would refuse his invitation! Through that box something amounting to £500 went to missionary work. And more recently, after the death of Blokie £70 trickled in for the Aberfan disaster fund "in memory of Blokie". While he was alive gifts of money were sent regularly to the WEC headquarters for Winnie's work, and the receipts would come back with the acknowledgement "Received from Blokie the little Crusader". Many of Winnie's letters to Briallen were acknowledgements of these gifts, telling how they had helped to provide medicines and pay for the food for the boarding school girls.

Blokie's first performance for Winnie was during her 1955

furlough. He sang "*Sospan Fach*" (Little Saucepan) and then said "God bless Winnie in Congo. *Salamu kwa Devi ku Congo*." (Greetings to David in the Congo.) "Please put a penny in the box." The tears were streaming down Winnie's face when he finished. She put her head on his cage and said, "In Elijah's time God sent ravens to feed him. Now God is using a budgie in Wales to feed the children in Congo."

Other friends that Winnie held dear were Briallen's friends also. Briallen introduced her to some of her fellow sufferers at the Royal Hospital and Home for Incurables in Putney, London. Winnie was able to pay them a very brief visit, but brief though it was, it brought the ladies and Winnie together in a close bond.

One of the ladies recalls, "We only had Winnie with us for less than an hour, but what a time of real happiness and blessing that was. She was all quietness and confidence. Sometimes when church friends come we feel awkward when they ask if they can read and pray with us in a crowded room, but with Winnie there was such a sense of peace that there was no embarrassment. What a wonderful woman to make friends in just over half an hour!" When Winnie returned to the Congo the ladies wrote to her every week until they were assured that letters could no longer reach her in her captivity. They also supported her work financially at great personal cost.

In July 1961 Winnie was all set for returning to the Congo. A valedictory service was held for her at Coedpoeth, and a recording made at this service gives an impression of Winnie's outspokenness and her intense love of the Congolese. "I am going to give you an illustration of the Church of Christ in Congo. It is a wonderful Church. I might even dare to say that it is a much better Church than the Church in this land. By this I am not talking about bricks and mortar. We are the Living Church: I am part of the Living Church, you are part of the Living Church. We who have been redeemed by the blood of the Lamb are part of it – and there is another part of it out there in the Congo. That Church has been founded on the Word of God.

"I go into homes in this land but do I ever see the Bible? Very, very rarely do I see it in a prominent place. The Bible is a hidden book. There in the Congo the Bible is a book that they love. The Bible is a book that is fingered, that is dirty and greasy because those dear people haven't their wash basins and their soap; they haven't the money to buy them, and we see their Bibles and they are dirty. Very often the children will get hold of them and they play with them. Their parents will see them and will smack them because they have the Bible, the precious Book.

"When these dear people travel, they don't have changes of clothing, they don't have all sorts of luggage with them, but one thing they *do* have is their part of the Living Church, this book, and it must go with them.

"If they are getting old they also have their glasses with them. These are their reading glasses and if they happen to break these glasses it sorrows them. Why? Because they cannot read the newspaper or some of the secular magazines that one sees on the bookstalls these days? No. They are upset, they are heart-broken because, as they say, 'What am I going to do about the Word? How shall I be able to read the Word?' The Bible is wonderful to them, it is their food and drink. One day an old woman came to me saying, 'I have broken my glasses. What am I going to do? I am not able to read the Word?' I tried to patch up her glasses until she was able to get some others . . .

"This is the thing, friends, which has made the Church of Christ in Congo a stable Church, a valiant Church, a triumphant Church. It is founded on the Book."

Another incident sums up her dedication as she faced the return to troubled Congo. Saying goodbye to friends in Manchester, Mr and Mrs Tilbrook, Winnie paused after the usual farewells and came back up the path to Mrs Tilbrook.

"Frances, there is only one thing I want. Only one thing I really long for. It is 'that I might know Him.' "

A few days after the meeting in Coedpoeth Winnie was back in London preparing for her flight to Congo. She seemed apprehensive and one of the missionaries at headquarters asked her if she really believed it was the Lord's time for her return.

"I must go back. This is the will of the Lord for me," Winnie replied with conviction.

When it came to packing Winnie remembered her "dear people" in the Congo, especially their need of reading glasses. Going by air restricted her to twenty kilograms of luggage, but she kept her personal things to a minimum so that she could take as many pairs of second-hand spectacles as possible.

The missionary who saw Winnie off at the air terminal recalls, "Her whole thought seemed to be about the Africans, especially those at Opienge. She was grieved because she had to leave some pairs of glasses behind. As hand luggage on the plane she had her big Swahili Bible and out of her carry-all were sticking numerous spectacle cases!

"We took her to the air terminal and as the man weighed her in he did not count her hand luggage (the carry-all overflowing with spectacles), so she was not up to full weight! She was quite upset about it and if there had been time I believe she would have gone back to HQ to collect the spectacles she had had to leave behind! Eventually she got on the bus for the airport, carrying her precious load. We waved goodbye to her as she sat alone in the bus looking sad as she left."

8

"I WANT TO BURN OUT"

If Winnie was sad at saying goodbye to her friends in London she certainly revived before she arrived on Congo soil again on July 9th 1961. Her long journey restored her as she saw God's hand protecting her. Before leaving home she had been assured that the Lord was going before her to prepare the way, and she had needed that assurance. To arrive alone in East Africa and then drive the long, dangerous road of nearly seven hundred miles through Kenya and Uganda into Congo was no easy matter in those unpredictable days. But she was sure of God and knew she did not travel alone.

Writing to a friend later she said: "Two days after arrival in Kampala saw me on the road for Congo, some missionary friends having kindly looked after my car for me during my stay in England. I travelled the first 160 miles in the company of a Rwanda Christian and his daughter. He was a real man of God and it was he who translated for Billy Graham when he was here in Africa last year.

"The next day I arrived at the Congo border. I had no re-entry permit and so had to look entirely to God to get me through the customs. This He did in His own wonderful way, and my heart simply wells up in praise to Him as I see how He abundantly fulfilled His promise in going before to prepare the way."

Winnie had to wait twenty-four hours to obtain the permit. During that time she received a message that Jim Grainger from Ibambi had gone to Kampala, and that if she waited he would be back soon, so they could travel together the rest of the way. This was remarkable, because the letters Winnie had sent to warn him of her arrival had not reached their destination.

"This caused my heart to rejoice more than ever," she continued, "for not only would I have someone with whom to travel but also God was fulfilling His word to me. Hallelujah!

"And so we started our journey into Congo. I really felt like doing as some of the Hebrews did when they arrived in Israel. They kissed the blessed ground!

"It was interesting to see the reaction of the Congolese as we motored in. We received a wonderful welcome wherever we went, the people shouting such words as 'Hallelujah', 'Welcome', 'Greetings'. Then when we arrived at our first WEC station they came running to us, saying with delight, 'Are we dreaming? Are we seeing things?,' because no one knew I was coming. It was a tremendous surprise to the Congolese and missionaries alike."

Pastor Jonas Danga was the first to meet Winnie as she got out of the car, and they exchanged greetings. "If trouble and persecution come again I shall not leave," Winnie said to him. "I shall stay even if it means death."

At Ibambi headquarters there was much discussion concerning Winnie's future sphere of service. There was no doubt in her mind: Opienge was again unstaffed by missionaries and she wanted to return there. The leader and committee hesitated to send her, because conditions were still precarious and there was no missionary available to go with her. She was asked to spend some time on another station and to evangelize the villages around.

Winnie went but was very restless. She confided to one colleague, "If I do not get back to Opienge I shall be ill." But she was not idle, as she reported: "Last Sunday I went into the bush to hold Sunday Schools: lots of children gathered, also adults. We had the great joy of seeing five girls coming to the Lord, and one woman asked for prayer because of her tongue, which she felt was an offence to God. Such a lovely touch from God, to give these souls so soon after returning to Congo.

"On Saturday we went to the shopping centre armed with literature, phonograph, tracts and a table. We had a wonderful reception. We played the gospel records (graciously given by Gospel Recordings) in the tribal languages and sold gospels and small books for a nominal sum. Lots of pygmies brought literature too."

At last it was decided that Winnie should pay a three and a half weeks' visit to Opienge with Daisy Kingdon in order to report on the safety of the situation.

Daisy Kingdon says, "We had an uneventful journey down. As we neared Opienge there were frequent stops so that the folk could greet her. She was greatly loved and was given such hugs and handshakes, especially by the Walumbi.

"Our evening walks there were frequently interrupted to talk to one person or another about the Lord. She was a great soul-winner. She was also a courageous soul. She drove to Bafwasende through the night to take a woman in labour to the hospital, and she also took a trip to Stanleyville in those troubled days."

Winnie gives her version of the welcome at Opienge in a letter to Briallen. "At last I have arrived in Opienge the Beloved. What a tremendous welcome we had! The nearby villagers had heard that we were expected that day and so there was a full turn-out as they heard the roar of the car coming from some distance away. The silencer had been damaged on the bad road!

"They came dancing and singing towards us waving branches of coloured bushes in their hands. Certainly there was no sign of our not being wanted. And when we arrived at the station the noise was deafening. Excitement was high, with everyone talking together . . . There is just one dark spot in the picture which clouds all our hearts when we think of it, and that is that I am here just for a three week's visit, there being no personnel to stay with us permanently. The joy leaves us somewhat when we think of my leaving again. It is almost unthinkable."

During that short time she did all she could for the people. The precious spectacles were brought out of the famous carry-all and put to good use. She wrote: "Since coming here I have been emptying my boxes in an effort to help the folks a little. Their gratitude knows no bounds. I have also been able to help them with spectacles. I told the friends at home about the need and so I was able to bring with me quite a number of pairs: old ones which I had tested and checked before coming, and some new ones also. They are simply delighted."

She could not speak highly enough of the Opienge Christians. "The faithfulness of the Christians has been wonderful. They are absolutely irreproachable. They have worked and endured. Their poverty has been very great but God has blessed them and caused them to overcome. The testimony of everyone around is that our people have been faithful and that they have carried on just the same as when the missionaries were here. Isn't that wonderful? Our God is blessing them.

"The things in my house are intact, too. Nothing is missing as far as I can see; everyone has been most faithful. Indeed one praises the work of Calvary when one sees what God has done for our Christians here. His work in the hearts of unlearned men is something that truly magnifies God's Son.

"It is evident that it is not the missionary who has built the Church, else it would have toppled with the going of the missionary. But the building is of God and so the Church has withstood the fiery darts of the enemy. Glory to His name!"

The Opienge Church well deserved her praise. It was, and is, one of the poorest Churches. The people are agriculturalists and depend on the markets for the sale of their cotton, rice and peanuts in order to get money. The soil is very poor and harvests are not dependable. Add to this, destruction by wild animals, economic instability making the markets irregular, and the treacherous state of the road holding up transport indefinitely. There have been times when the Opienge Church workers received no remuneration whatsoever for six to nine months a year. And when there was a little money there was certainly no back pay. It was, for the pastors, evangelists and others, a case of serving the Church there literally "for the love of God". They were servants of the Church like their "Mademoiselle", and not hirelings. It was not surprising that they could not be "bought" when facing the ugly threats of the Simbas. They had learnt to die to self long before they faced the knives and guns of the rebels.

But Winnie had to return to Ibambi as arranged. She immediately started to agitate to get back to Opienge. Writing to a relative she said: "I am supposed to wait for a companion to go there with me, but as it seems there is no one (we are frightfully short staffed) I trust that permission will be given for me to go alone. I am straining at the leash to get back there." And two months after arriving back in the Congo she was able to write: "You will rejoice with me to hear that I am now back at my old station, serving the Lord in the centre of His divine will. Oh, what joy this brings; it is truly past expression. I am simply thrilled to be back at Opienge, for I know this is where God wants me."

In the light of future events Winnie's deep conviction that God wanted her at Opienge is the more remarkable. She continued in the same letter: "The pressure on my spirit to get back here, alone if necessary, was tremendous. So much so that when I was here for a three weeks' visit (to see how safe it was) I told the sorrowful folk that I would soon be back. That gave me some courage and them too! So I prevailed upon our Acting Field Leader to allow me to return here alone, which he reluctantly did." And she adds: "I am the only white woman at Opienge, the nearest being a hundred miles away at the Unevangelized Fields Mission station at Boyulu. The peace and joy of being in the place of God's choosing for me is simply great . . .

"On the station my welcome is absolutely one hundred per cent . . . They want the missionaries and they realize that they need us. They appreciate every bit of help they can get from me and I am more than willing to give it – their servant for Christ's sake. Pastor Alieni Paul asked me to take the morning meetings (every morning at 6.30) and I am taking them through Genesis.

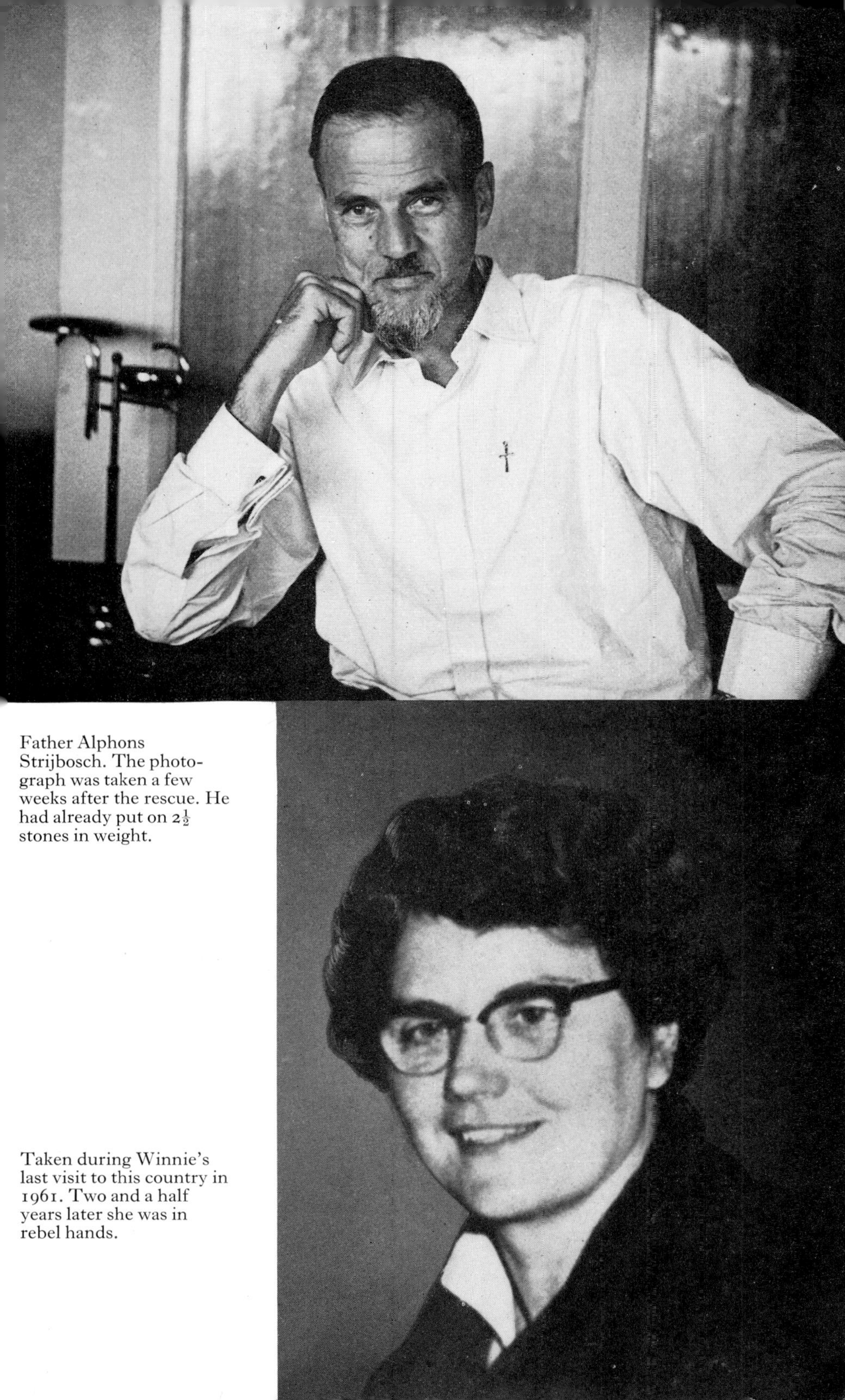

Father Alphons Strijbosch. The photograph was taken a few weeks after the rescue. He had already put on $2\frac{1}{2}$ stones in weight.

Taken during Winnie's last visit to this country in 1961. Two and a half years later she was in rebel hands.

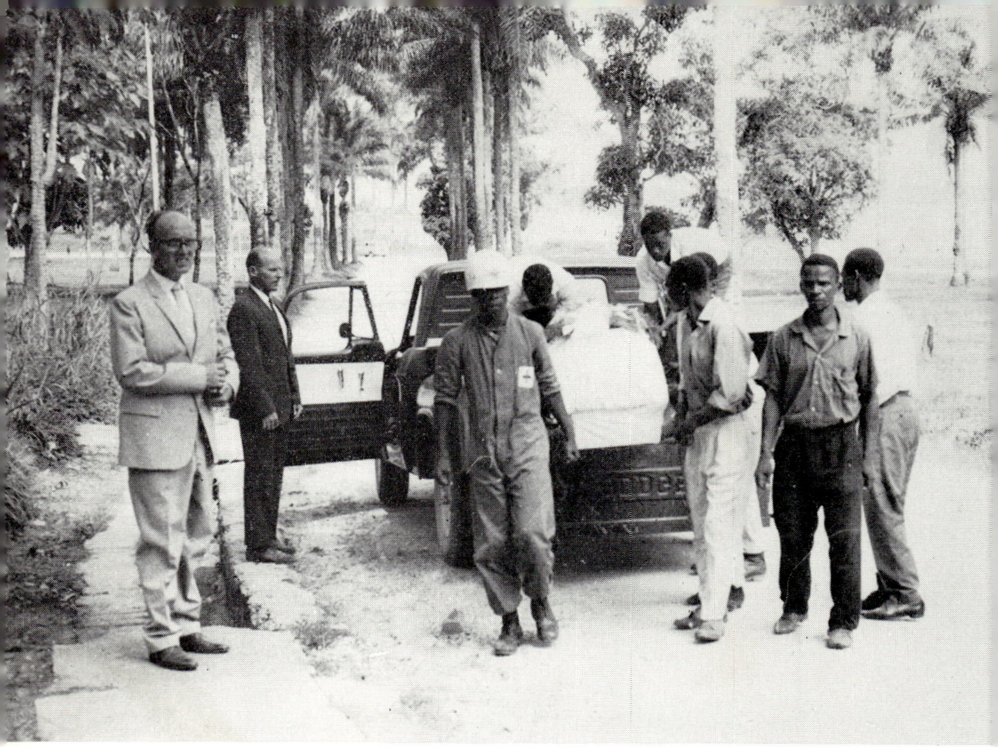

The coffin is carried to the BMS church, Kisangani, under the supervision of the Rev. Bill Gilvear. In the background is the great Congo River.

Winnie's day of triumph. "I have finished the work which Thou gavest me to do." "Christ shall be magnified in my body, whether it be by life, or by death."

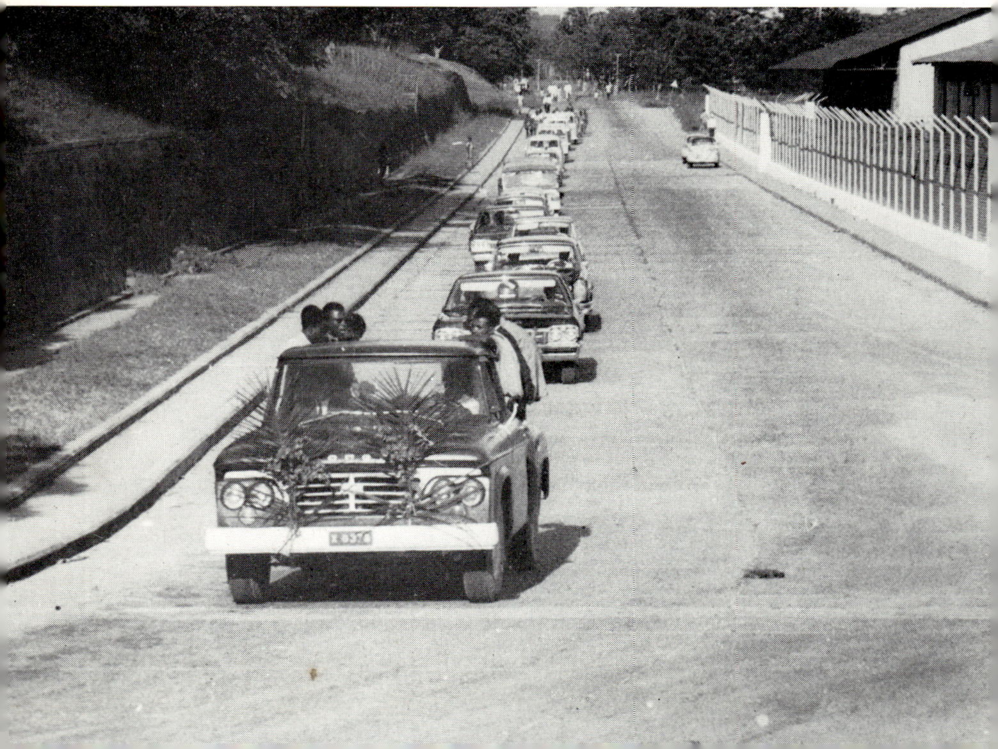

They simply drink in the teaching – they are thrilled with it; they say it consumes them and that God has brought me back to give them this teaching . . . You can see that their hunger for the things of the Spirit is keen and God is blessing."

As Winnie had realized, it had not only been her own pressing to return that had got her to Opienge again. The Congolese too had written strong appeals to the leader and committee asking them to allow their "Mademoiselle" to come back. They agreed to protect her and claimed that no one would touch Winnie except over their dead bodies. True to their word, the local Christians arranged a bodyguard for Winnie and when she did get back she was always shadowed by this guard, although she was unaware of it at first. What she did find was that Saboni and his wife Ana had been delegated to sleep in her house, Winnie upstairs and the couple downstairs. Many times in later months they risked their lives to protect their friend.

Winnie still had her Opel car, which had brought her back into the Congo, but she was finding it an increasing trial. It was low built, designed for level macadam roads, and was most unsuitable for the Opienge road. Huge trucks transporting rice from the Opienge rice factory travelled along it to the main Stanleyville road. The great wheels ploughed deep furrows both sides of the narrow road, leaving a high crown in the middle. The Opel was often left straddled on this crown, front wheels spinning, as the front of the car was lifted off the ground. Added to this, the road was no longer kept in repair since the closure of the Angumu gold mines after Independence, and the car suffered constant damage. On one occasion a rock cut through the car's steel protection plate and the sump box. Winnie wrote of another journey, "The other day my car broke down about eleven miles away from Opienge and the teacher who was with me ran all the way back to the mission to get help. He made the journey up and down dreadful hills in one and a half hours. What an achievement along such roads! The two Catholic priests came out to help me. We got back about 11.30 pm."

These breakdowns were all the more serious as there was no

garage within hundreds of miles. The Greek trader, the Roman Catholic priests and the Belgian official (when in residence) were all wonderfully kind to her. But there were times when the car was held up for weeks and even months until repairs could be made or parts obtained from Stanleyville. Winnie did not mention these incidents much but the final blow she did confide to a friend: "I don't know if I told you that my car has been damaged on one of the dreadful bridges. The local State workers have no nails to nail down the planks, so when the car touches them the planks go flying. This happened to me the other Sunday and a plank penetrated the radiator of my car.

"I had to be towed in and we are still trying to find a new radiator or even a second hand one, or perhaps get the damaged one repaired."

This incident spotlights the unbeatable spirit of this lonely woman. She constantly faced the possibility of a car breakdown on one of the most trying roads in the densest forest in the Congo, but she still desperately wanted to be mobile, travelling that road. Now, without the Opel, she felt her work was hampered and wrote to her friends at the Royal Hospital, Putney: "It seems almost impossible to get the car radiator repaired or to buy a new one. Being without a vehicle here in the bush is no fun. One man has already died of a strangulated hernia because I had no car to transport him to hospital."

A month or so later Winnie made a further desperate attempt to get the car repaired. She managed to get it to Stanleyville, where she stayed for a few days, standing over the job until she had succeeded in getting the Opel roadworthy once more. "At the moment I am in Stanleyville," she wrote, "having come here for a few days with my car for repairs. I was also in here a month ago for the same purpose but they didn't make a good job of it and so I have come all this way again: about six hundred miles the round trip.

"It is indeed pathetic to see Stanleyville, and compare what it used to be like with what it is now. The shops are empty or closed and all I was able to buy in the grocery line were two packets of ground tapioca with weevils (!) and two tiny bottles of onion essence . . . Matches are three shillings a box. One wonders just what will happen. The chemist said that he hadn't a single antibiotic in the shop, that penicillin had risen in price by three hundred per cent and that soon he would be selling the shop furniture. Tragic indeed!"

The day after Winnie left Stanleyville with her repaired car, further disturbances broke out in the town. She was fortunate to escape the fighting and plundering, and away at Opienge her work continued as usual. The only problem was of communication. "The mails are very irregular," she wrote. "I go for weeks without letters, so when they do arrive it is a 'Red Letter Day'! To take the post I have to depend mostly on African drivers who come here to fetch rice from the factory. Occasionally I have to send a man to do business for me at the post office. He has to walk ninety miles there and back, although he does all in his power to get a lift."

So she carried on her medical and spiritual ministry on her remote station, with hardly a reference in her letters to loneliness or homesickness. Indeed, her life was fully taken up with her African family. The boy "wee David", whom she had bottle-fed and cared for since Nebobongo days, often figured in her letters. "Young David, whom I have living with me, is full of life and keeps me lively. He loves to imitate people and last night he had us in stitches as he took off to the 'T' some people whom we know. He is very happy with me and can be very naughty too, but then, he is a boy and not an angel. At the moment he is ill, so I am giving him tonics to try to build him up – but taking medicines is not one of his strong points!" Other children gave her pleasure too. "At the moment I have a motor manufacturing company at the side of my house. The children, ten-year-olds, are pretending to make huge lorries complete with engines. The racket is sometimes excruciating as they sound the horn and make all the accompanying noises of a heavily loaded lorry stuck in the mud and trying to get out!! I have just been out taking their photos."

Some of her letters at this time mention her health. Since Nebobongo, migraine headaches had troubled her occasionally and she sometimes found the heat trying, but she now speaks of malaria as the main problem. Food parcels from Briallen Thomas arrived at just the right moment during these bad spells. "I have been in bed with malaria and it has left me pretty washed out," Winnie wrote. "I was still bedridden two days ago, and beginning to feel ravenously hungry all of a sudden, for I hadn't eaten for days. Then your lovely parcel arrived perfectly intact! My! how can I begin to thank you! It was like something dropped from Heaven – as indeed it was. I had just got one spoonful of tea left with no hopes of getting any more at present, and then God sent me two and a half pounds of it. I opened a tin of fruit immediately and it was good . . . I was in Stanleyville recently and the only thing I was able to buy in the stores was a packet of biscuits which when opened were mouldy, so I took them back and had my money returned."

Later Winnie was down with 'flu and again a parcel arrived. She wrote to the friends in Penydarren and the Royal Hospital, Putney: "Since Sunday (this is Friday) I have been longing to write to you but I have been ill with the 'flu. The day after the 'flu hit me, Sunday, your parcel arrived."

By the end of 1962 the roads had become so bad that Winnie could no longer use the Opel. "If I take the car I can never be sure that I shall be able to return, as the mud in parts is eighteen inches deep." So she sold the car to a man who could use it on the better roads in and nearer the towns. Being without a vehicle troubled her greatly, for she was not able to work as she wished. One instance was when a band of African volunteer missionaries undertook a journey to a distant tribe. "There are two couples with their families ready to go down south as missionaries to another tribe. Because I now have no car and will not have the honour of transporting them, they will have to take the cross country route through bush, forest, mountain and rivers. It is a really dreadful journey of about 350 miles and one of the women is pregnant. They will have to carry all their possessions on their backs. They do this in response to the command 'Go Ye'."

It is not surprising that Winnie began to make enquiries as to the best type of vehicle to have for her work. Her previous experience had taught her some hard lessons. She was told that a Land-Rover with a diesel engine would suit her purpose best and from then on her letters were full of plans for obtaining such a vehicle.

First of all, she approached the United Nations representatives at Stanleyville, asking their help in ordering a Land-Rover. When they replied that these were unobtainable in Congo but there was an order in for jeeps, Winnie immediately tried for permission to order a jeep. Letters were sent to government officials, visits were paid to the right departments, but without success. Finally she was driven to consider buying a Land-Rover from Britain and having it sent out to her via Mombasa.

In her efforts to get the car she deprived herself of everything she considered non-essential in order to build up a fund to pay for it. To her Penydarren friends she wrote: "Now please do ease off on those parcels, Briallen dear. They are so expensive to send. Please let it stay at that for a while. You asked if I would rather receive things in kind instead of money which you send from time to time. I would say 'No', as the money is precious ammunition, whereas the contents of your parcels, although tremendously appreciated, are to me luxuries, things I can do without. The money is vital . . . One comes to look on all food, apart from the bare essentials, as luxuries and it is surprising how easily one can do without them."

She closed another letter, "Dinner is about ready. These days I am eating elephant meat; it is surprising how nice it is! I was told that I would never be able to eat it unless it was the trunk, but whatever part I've got (and it's not the trunk) it is quite tender." It was obvious that Winnie was learning to make do with what little meat came her way. Perhaps her gift for creating something out of nothing was still with her, as the next extract suggests: "I had a joint of meat for dinner today and it was very good indeed. I usually cut up the meat into small cutlets to make it last longer but this was a gift that I received last night. A friend of mine whose baby I have treated for a bad burn gave me a leg of an animal he had caught in his trap. Also another friend sent me the hind leg of a little deer yesterday evening, but as I already had one leg in the oven, I gave it to the evangelist and his wife who live in my house with me in order to keep me company and guard me from danger. They were very thrilled."

The situation in the Congo did not improve. In April 1963 she wrote: "The food situation is still precarious here. Often we have no flour, sugar, milk and other necessities. The people who visit us from time to time in Opienge (Belgian officials and Greeks) are amazed when I tell them that I am so happy – I think they must look on me as a curio." In July she commented: "The priests are on furlough, two Greeks are away in Stanleyville and have been for about a month now, and the three remaining Greeks are going there tomorrow. I shall be the only European in this region for the time being."

Undaunted, she continued her ministry of self-giving for the people she loved. In August she mentioned in a letter the sense of urgency that kept her at her post rejoicing. "My thoughts are always on 'That Great Day'; and because of it I cannot allow myself to let up. These people are under-privileged, under-nourished, under-clothed and under-everything. I consider it a tremendous privilege to serve Christ and them. Indeed there is nothing more gloriously satisfying in life than to give oneself for others, and out here one has plenty of chances for doing so if one is alive to the opportunities."

Deprived of so much that people in Europe look upon as essential to happiness and deprived, in particular, of fellowship with her colleagues, she found that real happiness did not depend on material comforts. Very little reference is made to her own needs except to assure her friends that she is safe and content. Rather her letters were full of news of people, and of the further spread of the gospel at Opienge.

Gradually her fund towards a Land-Rover was built up. She

was disappointed to hear from the British Consul in Leopoldville that it was impossible to buy a car in the Congo with Congolese money: it would have to be paid for in foreign currency. This meant arranging for the money to be transferred to England and she found that it would lose one third of its value. But encouragement came when she heard of a gift of £300 towards buying a car, from a young woman in Britain who was going into Bible college shortly. And Winnie was able to write to Briallen: "There is also £10 from a widow with three children; she works during the day to keep them in school. My, what sacrifices you and the friends around Penydarren, RH and HI and others are making . . . I think when the Land-Rover arrives I will call it 'Blokie'!"

Winnie was quick to note these sacrifices, yet did not seem to recognize the sacrifice she was making. On April 8th 1964, just four months before the curtain of silence fell, she wrote to a young woman who felt called to serve God in the Congo: "How delighted I am that I gave my life to Him when I was young. I still give my life to Him as almost daily I repeat my vows of full dedication to Him, telling Him that my hands and feet and strength are all His, to do with them just as He wills. A great privilege and a great joy. Indeed if I had my life all over again I would choose no other way . . . I don't want to rot out, I want to burn out for Him."

Winnie knew nothing of the approaching peril when she wrote this. She continued: "About a fortnight ago I received a letter from some friends in Wales asking me what they had to do to get a Land-Rover despatched to me! I can't express to you how delighted I was . . . So I shall have a Land-Rover with a diesel engine by about July."

Her hopes ran high. In every letter she talked of the vehicle which would enable her to travel that awful road, and which would help her work of saving lives. "The roads are worse than ever and now it is the rainy season," she commented. "A Land-Rover, being a four-wheel drive, is the answer to these roads."

But in June her enthusiasm and hopes were checked. "I

received a letter from the friends who are interested in helping me purchase a Land-Rover. To say that I was shocked and disappointed at the news that a Land-Rover could not be delivered to the boat before December is to put it mildly. I had no idea that these vehicles were so difficult to obtain and that there would be a waiting list. I had thought my only barrier was the money."

In that same letter Winnie talked of other disturbing items of news. "Yesterday I heard that Mulele, the rebel who was trained in China and is causing so much trouble at the moment in Bukavu, has 'promised' to come to Stanleyville this month. He fights his wars with insects – so they say – such as stinging ants and hornets, etc. and it seems that he is very successful. One would think it devilish, if all we hear was true, but it may not be of course. Continue to pray for us . . ."

Thinking of her friends and relatives at home who might be distressed at the news of fresh unrest in the Congo, she wrote: "I can asssure you that there is no need to worry about me, as I I am perfectly all right, very happy in the Lord and in His blessed service. It delights me to serve the Lord and I never tire of the wonder of it – a servant of the King of Kings."

These were not empty words. Winnie meant them deeply and mentions in the same vein her longing for "fruit, fruit, fruit, lasting fruit. That is my prayer these days, that souls might be born from above and become real workers for Him."

The work was developing and the new hospital at Opienge was now a reality. Winnie wrote: "The population appreciates it very much. So now we have a dispensary, a maternity and a hospital, together with a new primary school and qualified teachers. I am also supporting some of the children in secondary school.

"So apart from the preaching of the gospel of Jesus we give the people that which is necessary for life also. We distribute milk and food which we obtain from relief organizations, and when I receive parcels of clothes I distribute these."

July 1964 was the date fixed for the WEC mission conference

at Ibambi Head Station. Winnie did not want to go because it meant leaving her people again for a couple of weeks. But arrangements were made for a truck to pick her up and she agreed to attend.

The conference was a milestone in the mission's work in Congo. It was there the missionaries confirmed the rightness of their action taken some years previously, when they had handed over the Church affairs to the Africans. Now the Africans gave abundant proof of their ability, sense of responsibility and maturity.

The conference was also a milestone for other reasons. Some of the missionaries present were to be killed within the next four months and Winnie herself was to be shut off behind a sinister Simba curtain of silence for nearly three years. The silence was broken just intermittently by rumours that she was alive.

I and the others who were present at that conference remember how Winnie urged that we missionaries should split up more often in order to have meals with the Africans, and how she responded when the situation at Opienge was examined. We wanted her to remain around Ibambi for a couple of months to wait for an amelioration of the unrest; also, a new missionary was soon to leave Britain for the Congo. This would make changes possible and so provide Winnie with a companion. Winnie got to her feet in the meeting and quietly but firmly said, "I know God is with me. I must go back to Opienge."

Just before coming to the conference Winnie had written in a letter: "It will be strange talking English again. I use only Swahili and French here." But if she felt any strangeness it soon vanished and one of the missionaries at the conference commented, "Winnie has been for some time by herself at Opienge. Some of us feared what the reaction would be after so long without company – but she was just full of the joy of the Lord."

Thursday July 16th was the day for dispersing. As Winnie had no transport Arthur Scott offered to take her back to

Opienge. He recalls: "Just before 6 am we said our farewells. We were soon loaded in the pick-up van with the African delegates who had come from Opienge.

"The route was a familiar one. Our first stop was Wamba, about fifty miles from Ibambi. Then Bafwapoka, the birthplace of 'wee David'. Here we met the relatives of the lad and while we ate our picnic lunch the future of David was discussed. In true African style they entered into a palaver. Wisely Winnie left the family to make the decision. David wanted to return with Winnie. Later they came to tell us that it was their wish for David to remain with her.

"We journeyed on another fifteen miles and stopped to have fellowship with a grand unpaid evangelist, Sali; it was an enjoyable time together. Then on through Bafwasende to Boyulu, where over a cup of tea with Mr and Mrs Chester Burke, we shared news. Here Winnie had her last contact with Protestant missionaries."

If only these places could speak what stories of torture and massacre and of victories through Christ they would tell! Wamba was the scene of the killing of Jim Rodger and Bill McChesney. Bafwasende was soon to be known all over the world as a place of death for many missionaries working with the Unevangelized Fields Mission. Boyulu yielded a similar story as Mrs Burke suffered and Chester Burke was killed.

Arthur Scott continues: "Another twenty miles further on we left the main road to begin the last stage of our journey to Opienge. Winnie had not said anything about the difficulties experienced on the outward journey until we were on this road. Now I was told that the sixty-five mile stretch had taken them from early morning until very late at night! In fact they only made it in the one day by the help of a tractor that towed them through the mud on the last stage of the journey.

"Our passage was smooth going, by comparison. Once we became bogged down, but with the help of the passengers we were soon on the road again. We edged our way over one of the bridges inch by inch, as most of the wood had broken away. For a safe journey along that unpredictable stretch of road we were grateful to God.

"As we travelled Winnie shared with me some of her problems and plans concerning the Church at Opienge. She spoke about how keen she was for some of her nurses to get further training. She wanted them to have the very best so that those to whom they ministered could receive the benefit of their added experience. Her interest in youth was evident from plans she had for her school teachers to share in further training schemes too. She had invited one missionary couple to come to Opienge for a short-term Bible school. She wanted to see the Church leaders encouraged and built up in the faith.

"In talking of the early morning meetings, she told me her Bible readings with the Christians were from the Book of Revelation. How far into the book they had reached before the Simbas came we do not know. I have often wondered if she had dealt with the 'great multitude' in chapter seven that had 'come out of great tribulation'.

"About 7 pm we passed the few shops at Opienge, turned left into the mission station and drove up to Winnie's house. News of her arrival soon spread and from all directions the Africans appeared and converged upon us. There was plenty of noise! Some were singing, others shouting their welcome, while all were pressing forward to shake her hand. Excitement continued for a long time but eventually we were able to sit down to a very welcome meal. The following morning my African evangelist companion and I said goodbye to Winnie and the Opienge Christians and began our homeward journey."

Arthur thought it would be but a few months before he saw Winnie again; he had offered to go to Mombasa to fetch the Land-Rover as soon as word came of its arrival there. The farewell was a happy one, with a wave of the hand and "God bless. See you soon with the Land-Rover."

"A few weeks later," Arthur continues, "Winnie sent me further details about the expected arrival in Mombasa of the car, and enclosed some blank cheques to cover my expenses to East Africa to collect it."

In her anxiety to have the vehicle Winnie had written to the Rover Company, explaining her predicament and appealing to them to get it to her at the earliest date possible. Writing on July 23rd, she said: "I returned from the conference a few days ago and found some mail awaiting me. In it was a letter from the Rover Company. They said they would have a Land-Rover ready for me, owing to my adverse circumstances, for delivery to the boat by September. Isn't it wonderful? They asked me for a reply by the 14th of this month but it was already the 17th when I received the letter. Such is mail in Congo today!"

"Won't it be a wonderful day when the long anticipated vehicle arrives? How very essential it is for the smooth running of the work. Praise God that His time is always best."

Winnie did not realize when she wrote that last sentence how it was to be proved in reality. If the car had arrived in July as Winnie had first hoped, it would have been seized, used and destroyed by the Simba rebels in the months that followed.

A few more letters came through telling of her work. On July 29th she wrote: "I have just come from the Women's Meeting, where there were a lot present. We start off with a reading class for those who don't know how to read. Then we have prayer, hymns, testimony and then prayer again – for Congo; the situation is really grave and it looks as though there will soon be widespread civil war. Then came the message given by one of the women. I was called out during this, to a dying child, but one thing I heard was, 'Look after your Christianity.'

"What a good, essential and very down-to-earth admonition! If we all looked after our Christianity I am quite sure that we would be different Christians and the world would be a different place."

There were four more letters from Winnie soon after, all dated July 31st 1964. We find in them great anticipation of the promised visit to Congo by Mr Len Moules, the International Secretary of WEC. "He will be coming in September and will be visiting us here at Opienge. We had feared that as we are so far off the main route we should be deprived of a visit, but no, he will stay with us two days.

"News of Congo is very disturbing, isn't it? The Lumumba party is very active . . . We have a lot of that party in our area. They have openly said that the first to suffer would be that State, then the people of God, then the rich. So there you are! However, for the moment all is quiet."

To her family (her father had married again) she wrote: "I am perfectly all right and safe. My folks concern themselves very much about my welfare and were saying just last night that they wanted another couple to sleep in my house, for my protection. I told them that there was no need whatsoever, and that Ana and Saboni who sleep in my house were sufficient. However, I promised them that if there should be trouble in the area another couple could come in."

Then, after some weeks of silence, one more letter addressed to her parents arrived in Coedpoeth. It was dated October 2nd 1964. Was it carried by native courier, or a friendly Simba perhaps, to be picked up by the Red Cross at Stanleyville? Winnie wrote; "It's a long time since I wrote you because there was no way of getting letters out of the country, or at least, out of this Province. However, I may be able to get this out by means of the Red Cross plane, which I hear will be coming in about a month's time. Here's hoping anyway!

"I am perfectly well and there is no need to worry about me. I have stayed in Opienge all through the crisis. It has been pretty grim. I shan't be able to give details as the letters may be censored. We've had no mail since the end of July. My typewriter is not working well as you may notice from the bad type.

"I am hoping that the Land-Rover company have *not* sent the car out to Mombasa, for I have no way of knowing anything, and if it is there I will have to pay storage for every day, which will come to a large amount. It is fortunate I do not have it here, for it would be mine no longer, as has happened to all the cars in the province.

"The Greeks are no longer here. The nearest white person is about one and a half miles away, where there are three priests. But I am perfectly safe and tremendously respected by the new army. Have not heard anything from any of our missionaries since the emergency; one supposes that all are well, but one doesn't know. However, I am told that the mail is beginning to pass again, so I shall have a try at sending some letters to the missionaries . . .

"David is well; he sends his love to you. He is still very nervous as we have had fearful experiences, but these last couple of days he is a little better . . ."

Obviously Winnie could not divulge very much in that letter. The following chapters will give some idea of the depth of meaning behind such phrases as "It has been pretty grim . . . My typewriter is not working well . . . We have had fearful experiences . . ."

During the two months between the writing of the last two letters things had been "pretty grim" indeed. It was surprising that the typewriter worked at all when, with all her other goods, it had been stolen and returned on more than one occasion. But the story of those weeks, and the months ahead, was to be shut up behind a Simba curtain of silence for almost three years.

9

SIMBA REVOLUTION

Compared with the upheaval at the time of Congo's independence in 1960, the Simba uprising of 1964 erupted, like a volcano, with terrifying suddenness. It not only threw the country into mad disorder; it let loose a ghastly flood of murder and torture so wild and widespread that it shook the world.

The communist-inspired Pierre Mulele had led a revolt in January 1964 in the Province of Kwilu. He had trained young men in secret camps, arming them with spears, bows and arrows and any old guns they could find, and preached to them a revived faith in witchcraft which, he said, would turn bullets to water. This gave rise to the cry soon to be heard in three-quarters of the Congo, "Mayi, mayi, Lumumba mayi." (Water water, Lumumba water.) "Mayi, mayi, Simba mayi. Mayi, mayi, Mulele mayi."

With almost incredible speed these Simbas (Lions) spread northwards from Kwilu Province and by the beginning of August, Stanleyville, Banalia and Buta were in their hands. After only five hours of fighting, Opienge was taken on August 14th.

Aiming further north, Mulele sent telegrams to Wamba and Paulis announcing his arrival. He did this to most towns and rarely failed to arrive on the day announced. In most cases the telegram struck such terror into the hearts of the soldiers defending the towns that they changed into civilian clothes and deserted. They had heard the wild stories of the power of Mulele and his incredibly savage treatment of his captives. To some areas Mulele had even sent chunks of human flesh with a note – "This is what is going to happen to you if you resist us!"

At Paulis, where my wife and I were based, the ground had been well prepared, as elsewhere, for Mulele's coming. All youth movements had been indoctrinated by secret agents. New political parties appeared almost every week. Teachers and civil servants had been for months without wages, while government officials made sure of their own pay and more. They lived in luxury while in the native towns many thousands of Congolese lived at starvation level. After the disturbances of 1960 many Belgians had not returned to the Congo, and others had returned to find disrupted plantations, mines or factories. This aggravated the unemployment situation and thousands of Africans were workless. Africans in their bush villages managed to live independently of wages and shops, but nearer civilization they depended on a wage to obtain food and clothing.

Into this seething cauldron of unrest moved the secret agents stirring up resentment by suggesting, "Let's overthrow the Government and set up another which will provide fairness all round." The hungry masses were ready for any revolution which promised them full stomachs.

A day or two after Mulele's telegram had arrived at Paulis my wife and I were some miles away preaching at an outlying church. While eating our lunch a car full of soldiers drove up. They were apparently fleeing from Paulis and demanded petrol from us for the car they had requisitioned. Only in the nick of time one of our Christians whispered, "There's a palm oil factory just a mile up the road." We told the soldiers we would go to the factory for petrol and, hastily filling our car with people, we drove off. Once they had the petrol the soldiers forced the half-caste driver of the car to drive on. Almost immediately another truck full of soldiers dashed by. The young Belgian at the wheel put his head out of the cab and yelled "I am being forced to take them to Niangara."

This was our first indication of the seriousness of the situation. As we returned to Paulis we discovered that with the desertion of the soldiers it had become the prey of plunderers. At last Mulele's "arrival" day came and he came with it. In all sorts of cars, pickups and trucks the rebels came, shooting their guns into the air to make their entrance known. In a matter

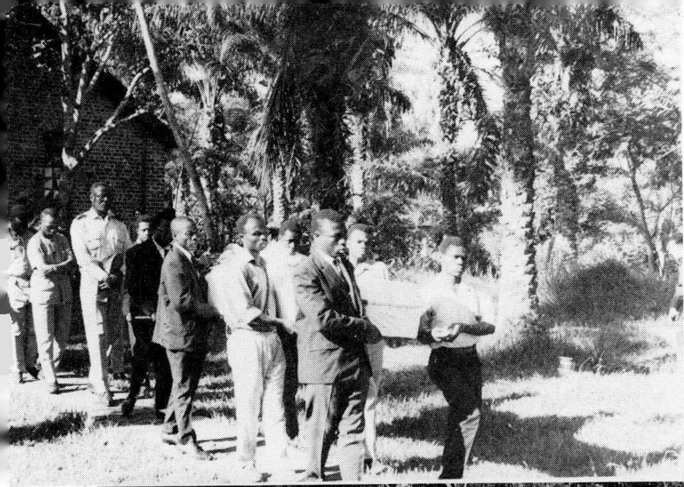

Immediately behind the coffin is the Governor of the Province (with the white stick) and General Tshinyama of the National Army.

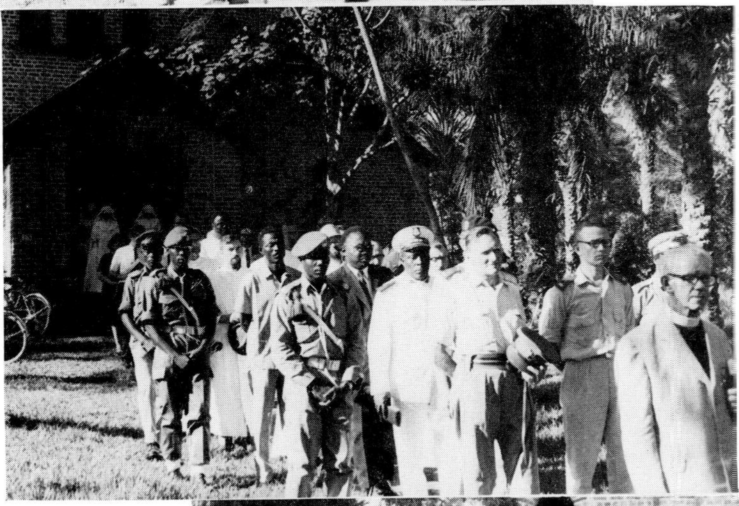

Leaving the church after the service. In the foreground, the Rev. G. Kerrigan and Colonel Brook Fox, Military Attaché, holding cap in hand.

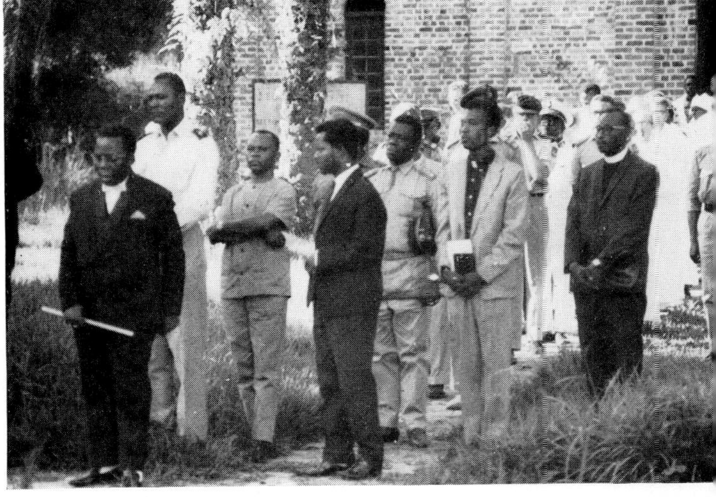

The Governor of the Province, General Tshinyama, members of the Salvation Army, Pastor Assani (UFM), priests and nuns of the Roman Catholic Church and civilians follow the coffin.

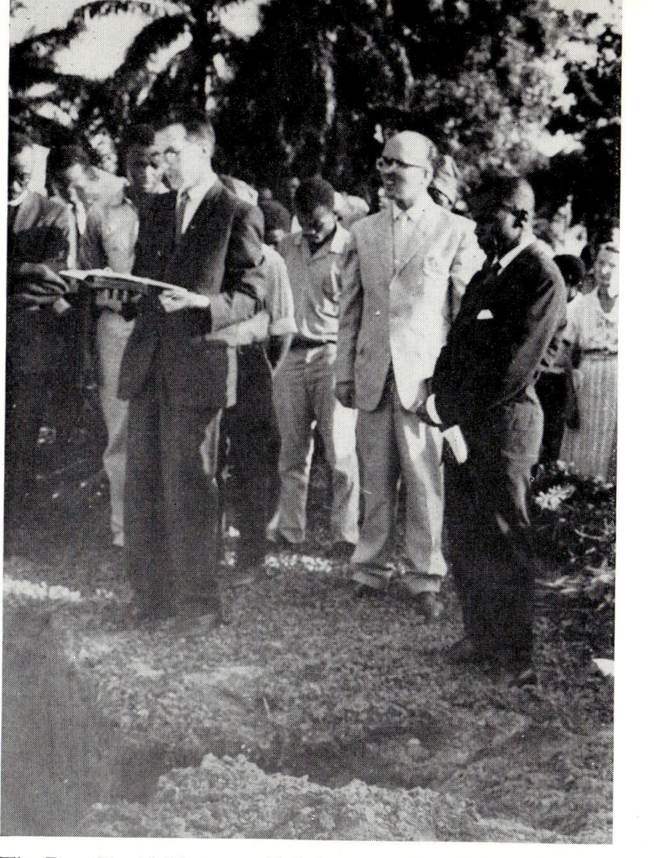

The Rev. David Claxton, officiating, was himself buried twelve days later, the victim of bandits. A double tragedy? No. Two seeds buried, assuring a harvest to the glory of God.

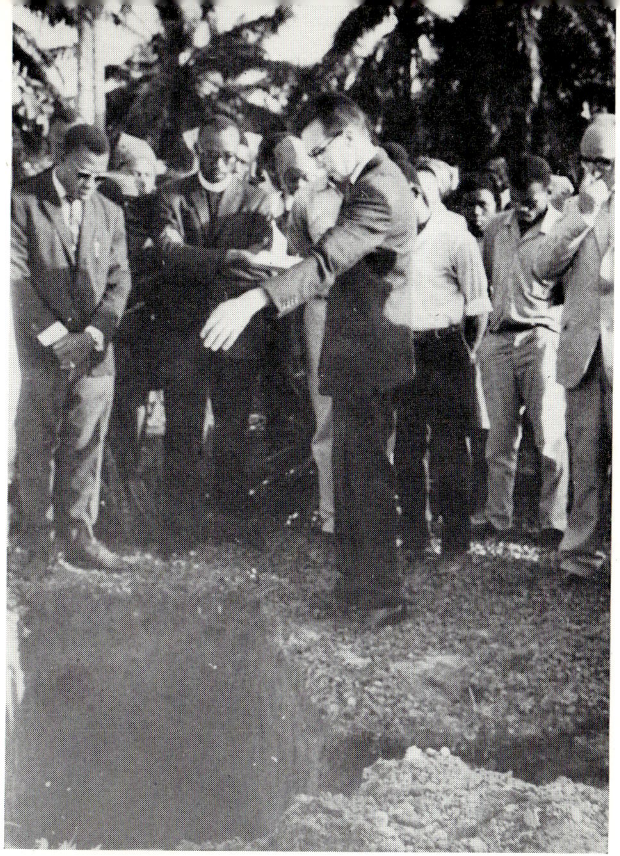

"If in this life only we have hope . . . we are of all men most miserable." But Winnie, "in sure hope of eternal life" has reached the other side.

of moments they were in complete charge of everything and the terror began. Every employee of the State was rounded up and liquidated. By the decision of a "People's Court" the rich, well-dressed, educated Africans were tortured and despatched. Within the first two weeks over two thousand Congolese were inhumanly tortured and killed near the flagstaff. Then the terror spread into the district.

But what of Winnie? There was not a breath of news. Nearly all the evacuated missionaries who reached their homeland felt there could be little possibility that she was still alive after the taking of Opienge

The first ray of hope came through a letter from Father Leon Mondry, one of the Roman Catholic priests working at Opienge. He was arrested and taken from Opienge on November 5th 1964, and he promised he would, if liberated, send news of Winnie to her family. This he did on his arrival in Belgium on December 3rd. So the news that Winnie was alive on November 5th was almost a month old when it reached her relatives.

Seven months of grim silence passed. Then on July 8th 1965 a telephone call came from the Foreign Office. The British Embassy in the Congo had received a letter from a Greek trader who had been in business at Opienge, but had escaped and was now at Stanleyville. He had written to say that some of his workers had reported that Miss Davies was alive and being cared for.

In October of the same year a report was sent from Stanleyville to the effect that Winnie had been moved from her remote station at Opienge to the rebel stronghold of Bafwasende. An attempt by the Congolese government forces to retake this town was heavily repulsed about that time.

A month later, on November 17th, the London Foreign Office informed the WEC in London that the Leopoldville Embassy had stated: "No attempt to rescue Winnie Davies can be made this year, due to heavy commitments at the Lake around the eastern border."

Nothing more was heard until April 25th 1966, five months later. A letter from Miss Margaret Hayes of the Unevangelized

Fields Mission included a letter which she had received from a priest in Holland. The priest stated that Winnie and a Dutch priest had been taken to Batama at Km 148 on the Stanleyville road, and were camped about ten kilometres from the main road in the bush. Some women who had escaped brought the news that Winnie and the priest were in good health but well guarded.

The tension was mounting now that it was certain Winnie was alive. Attempts to catch the rebels were made, but in October the news was that an army column reaching Batama had just missed them; the rebel general, aware of the approaching army, had moved away with forced marches into the deep forest of the Bomili area.

Three months of silence and agonizing suspense followed. On January 6th 1967 John and Del Gunningham wrote from Leopoldville: "This morning the Embassy rang to say that they have definite and reliable information that Winnie was seen alive on January 4th. She had been taken by 'the lions' to the area at the back of the UFM station at Maganga. The Embassy are wiring her next of kin to let them know that she is definitely alive. They hope that she will be handed over within the next few days. The rebel leader is said to be waiting for the best moment to surrender.

"We trust this is so. For the past month it has been circulated here that she has been killed and her body with that of a priest thrown into a disused church. A rebel colonel has been captured. It was he who murdered a nun at Isiro and gave orders to kill our missionaries at Wamba. He was going to do the same to more of his hostages when the Simbas turned on him and would not do the killings. He is now in jail at Isiro awaiting trial."

In February the WEC released a report that there was no likelihood of any rescue attempt being made for another four weeks. Colonel Fox, the British Military Attaché in Leopoldville, was doing a Trojan job trying to get the Congolese authorities to do something towards Winnie's release. The report stated: "The French-led commando unit based in

Stanleyville is not willing to go to Opienge until the bridges are rebuilt. The Belgian-led mercenaries in Lubutu are willing to walk to Opienge and rescue her, but this is nearly an impossible task because of the dreadful terrain–jungles, hills and no paths."

Nothing more was heard for two months. Then came another report confirming that Winnie was alive, being well treated and carrying on her nursing duties. "The one hardship she suffers along with the others is a shortage of food. It is thought that a Dutch priest is also a prisoner there."

The pressure was mounting, and moves were made to have Winnie rescued despite the unwillingness of the mercenaries to make the journey. Each time a heartening bit of news was received, it was promptly circulated to the various WEC centres and the many churches in Britain where people were praying for Winnie's release. All over the world her safety was the concern of WEC friends and meetings were held at home and abroad for specific prayer for her safety.

At last first-hand news of Winnie's captivity came through. On Sunday April 9th 1967 a Greek trader brought a letter from Pastor Alieni Paul to Dr Helen Roseveare at the Inter-Mission Medical Centre at Bunia. Alieni Paul had been in close contact with Winnie during 1964 and 1965 and had managed to escape from the forest on March 28th. He was at Bafwasende and pleaded with Dr Roseveare to visit him there. The letter was timely, as it coincided with plans already afoot for Helen Roseveare and Nurse Thompstone (UFM) to visit the area. The Greek trader assured them that the road was usable and the bridge over the Lindi River had been repaired, so they decided to set off immediately. Every inch of the car was packed with medicines, food, clothes and items of hardware for distribution to the needy people around Bafwasende.

The reunion with Pastor Alieni Paul was very touching, for he had been through a great deal. Before long Dr Roseveare was able to send home Pastor Alieni Paul's recollections of the arrival of the rebels at Opienge, and what followed. Slowly the curtain of silence was being lifted.

10

PASTOR ALIENI'S STORY

Alieni Paul was the first of the Walumbi to be set apart by the Church for the work of a pastor. Highly respected by the Christians and the native population, he naturally became a leader. During and after the "Independence" period he gave Winnie some heartaches because he seemed to be fostering an "Independence" spirit within the Church at Opienge, but it was only a passing phase and his consistent Christian example and his loyalty to Winnie showed his true worth.

With his daughter Priscilla and nephew Philbert, Pastor Alieni left the Ibambi Field Conference in July 1964 along with other Opienge Church representatives. Priscilla and Philbert were going to Opienge on their summer holidays from the Nebobongo nurses' training school. They wondered what lay ahead, as news filtered through of rebel victories to the south but as yet all seemed well.

They caught the bus to Bafwasende, hoping that from there Winnie, who was following with Arthur Scott in the mission car, would be able to take some of them part of the way to Opienge. At Bafwasende, on the east bank of the wide, fast-flowing River Lindi, the large, rickety bus stopped at the road fork. Sorting out their cases from the vast jumble of baskets, boxes, livestock and children piled up at the rear, they clambered down.

It was raining steadily from a grey sky and no one came out to help them. Reaching the evangelist's house, they settled down to wait on the verandah for the mission car. The last hundred mile stretch of the journey was the most difficult, as the road went south from the main Stanleyville road, deep into the wild mountainous forest around Opienge.

The next day Priscilla and Philbert, who had decided to hitch a lift home on their own, went to one of the Greek stores to see if they could find a car. Philbert was proudly wearing his Campaigner uniform with a row of badges on his right arm. Suddenly armed police surrounded the pair, struck Philbert over the head and roughly led him off to prison.

Nothing would persuade them that he was not a soldier. They took his belt and "lifeline" rank, and beat him, demanding his membership card of the MNC, the political party that had held undisputed sway in that area ever since Independence.

Philbert showed them his school pass to prove he was still a schoolboy and therefore forbidden to take part in politics, but they tore it up and just shouted abuse at him. After a night of this maltreatment in prison he was released. He and Priscilla set out at once towards Opienge, fearful at this hint of trouble to come.

They managed to get a lift from a Congolese chauffeur going to a large Belgian plantation thirty miles north of Opienge, and they walked the remaining distance. The road wound endlessly, crossing and recrossing by narrow two-plank bridges innumerable streams in deep valleys of virgin forest. Then, rising steeply, the road climbed the next line of hills, which were dotted with scattered villages and clearings newly planted with neat lines of cotton.

With relief they reached Opienge; all was quiet and peaceful. The grim experience at Bafwasende faded as they saw work going on as usual on the busy mission compound. Only on the further hilltop was there an unusual silence; all the children from the boys' school compound were scattered to their homes for the long summer holiday.

At the hospital centre it was "business as usual" and, after a week of visiting relatives, resting and helping her mother in the garden, Priscilla went to help Winnie with the medical work. Over the years Winnie had built up a thriving medical centre. There was a three-roomed hospital with some fourteen beds, a ten-bed maternity compound and a large out-patient dispensary where she saw some three thousand patients annually. It was not surprising, then, that she was sincerely loved by the Congolese. Patients came from all over the area to see her, attracted by her patience, kindliness, thoroughness and obvious concern for each individual. A nominal charge was made for their dispensary card, but few ever baulked at paying, knowing well that Winnie's careful examination, diagnosis and treatment of their condition was worth far more than the price of the card!

At Opienge *poste*, beside the handful of Greek stores served by four Greek families and many African shopkeepers, and the Roman Catholic community centre served by three European priests, there was a government dispensary. Although it was cheaper to go to this dispensary at the *poste*, few stopped there, preferring the extra five minutes' walk to the mission and Winnie's care.

On August 3rd, a fortnight after the return home from the Ibambi conference, news came over the radio of the Simba takeover of Kindu, south of Stanleyville. It looked as if Stanleyville was their next target in the great drive northwards.

The four Greeks and one of the priests came to Winnie.

"We're leaving at once for Stanleyville," they said anxiously. "Come with us. We cannot leave you alone here."

"No, no. I cannot leave again!" Winnie said. Her mind went back to 1960 with its rapid evacuation, fear and near panic, and the return later to the gentle rebuke of the Church: "Why did you leave us when we most needed your love and guidance and strength? Couldn't the Lord have cared for you, as well as for us?" No, she would not leave them again; she belonged here with them.

The Greeks pressed her to leave, but she said, "Give me till tomorrow," adding in an undertone, "but I'm sure I won't go."

She hastily called Pastor Alieni Paul and the evangelists who had gathered to hear a report of the Ibambi conference.

"War is coming," she said bluntly. "What do you want? Shall I leave or stay with you? If He chooses I die with you here."

They considered the matter for a week, praying and discussing the situation, but meanwhile Stanleyville was taken and the Greeks insisted on leaving immediately. The pastor and all the church elders said unanimously, "Go", but Winnie felt now the conviction in her heart that she must stay. "No," she replied, "I'm ready to suffer with you for Him. If it is really true that they are killing Christians, then I will die with you here."

Evangelist Saboni and his wife Ana, who were still staying with her, urged her to leave with the Greeks and other whites while there was time. But she felt more and more strongly God's quiet urging to stay. Finally the church elders agreed and quickly arranged to move into the station with their wives and families, so that everyone should be in one place when the day of reckoning arrived.

Patients and women poured in from all over the area, old and young, needy and grateful, all with one cry, "Don't leave us!" The station was filled with several hundred people camping in the compound, in the hospital, in the church and in every available home.

It was Friday August 14th. All morning the rain had poured down in torrents amidst thunder and lightning. After lunch, the clouds parted slightly and in the lull Winnie ran across to the hospital to see her patients. There was a deep stillness before the breaking of the fury of the next storm.

Like a moving forest of waving palm fronds, two trucks drove into the compound filled with soldiers stripped to the waist and garlanded with leaves. Grim faced, hard eyed, hatred in every line, they each had fur bands on head and wrists and gripped a rifle. They meant business and at the sight of them fear seized everyone. Hearts stopped in panic. It was suddenly hard to breathe.

"The Simbas arrived at Opienge on August 14th," says Pastor Alieni. "They quickly entered the mission and arrested Mademoiselle and me and made us stand together. They intended to kill us on the spot and prepared to throw their spears at us. I stood between them and Mademoiselle and said to her, 'Take hold of my belt, at my back.' She did so, but there were only the two of us amid a crowd of oppressors. They raised their spears to throw so I hastily pushed Mademoiselle backwards. One spear touched her hand but fell harmlessly to the ground. She escaped that first danger."

Alieni and Winnie were indeed alone. The Simbas' President had stridently demanded everyone's attention, telling them the Popular Army of the People had taken over. Everyone was to appear on parade the next day with their MNC card in hand. The soldiers left, but the hundreds gathered on the compound melted away. The station was deserted! Within an hour Winnie found herself alone with Pastor Alieni because only they had the necessary cards. All the others had fled to the forest in horror and fear.

Winnie, gathering up her handbag and identification papers, went to the Government offices, now "under new management". There she bought and signed for cards for the whole of her large family. Alieni set out into the forest in the evening, searching the people out and encouraging them as he distributed their membership cards for the new regime.

Next morning unruly rebel soldiers rushed to the mission to murder Winnie and Pastor Alieni. They shot at Winnie but the bullet passed through her dress, grazing her right hip. Alerted by others, the President arrived in time to stop further activity, and the Simba responsible was roughly tied up and beaten for touching the white lady without a proper trial. Then the President proceeded to make a detailed inspection of Winnie's house with coarse civility. No gun or transmitter having been found, money was demanded. She gave it to them unresistingly and at last they left. Moments later wild shouting and shooting was heard at the *poste*. Three policemen who had been tied up and thrown into prison had been murdered.

Two days later another crowd of soldiers mobbed the station and roughly grabbed Winnie and Pastor Alieni, driving them before them to the offices. The President of the Women's party had accused them. It was difficult to know of what. But it seemed to be the result of an old and deep-seated hatred, the working of a buried resentment. On one occasion Winnie had failed to attend the compulsory meeting of the Women's Party, being busily engaged with a difficult case in the maternity. This failure was chalked up against her as "adverse politics", linked to a belief that she also discouraged the wives of church elders from attending these political indoctrination classes.

Now the soldiers demanded to see Winnie and Alieni's membership cards. They showed them. Accusations were starting to flow when the President arrived and once more intervened on Winnie's behalf.

"Why bring her here?" he asked. "She has signed she is a *Congomani*, one of us. What more do you want?"

Alieni talked with them of Winnie's work and selfless love for the Congolese, her faith and goodness; and the President staunchly declared, "Let her be! We cannot kill our doctor!"

Alieni Paul recalls: "I was able to call the evangelists together. We talked to the Simbas and told them we would not allow them to take Mademoiselle away because we did not know what wrong thing she had done. So the Simbas decided to leave her for the time being."

Slowly an uneasy peace settled and work carried on quietly with little interference. Food was demanded periodically and they heard of various people in the area being beaten, or even killed. Fear lay heavy in the air, but they claimed God's peace and continued His work.

Then came November 24th when the National Army, aided by paratroopers, delivered Stanleyville from the rebels. Over the wireless came the details of the involved tragedy and triumph. A plea for the rebels to surrender followed – a plea for the raising of a white flag to show a willingness to welcome the National Army. The rebel adjutant at Opienge sought out Winnie at once, and a white flag was made and hoisted outside the government offices. All waited tense and hopeful.

Before any surrender became possible the rebel commander of the area, General Ngalu, heard of this act. In a blazing fury he sent a detachment of Simbas to tear down the flag and tie up and kill every Simba involved in this treasonable act.

The Adjutant, Jean Marie Nyambiamba, was the first one to be seized, but before he was shot he asked for time to talk with the white lady. His request granted, he talked with Winnie in the open courtyard before the hostile gaze of a growing crowd, and opened his heart to receive God's forgiveness of sin in Christ. He had been a good man, despite his strange allegiance to the rebel cause. Several times he had protected Winnie from the savagery of the soldiers and he had regularly attended the Opienge church, listening intently to the teaching. He had bought a Bible and talked with Winnie about his spiritual need and the way of salvation. Now, at the last, he publicly announced his faith in the living God and claimed His pardon.

Another who was killed at that time, Kwonga, was a complete contrast. He had several times troubled Winnie, even beating to death the son of a local chief who tried to protect her from his wickedness. He died in haughty silence, hardened to the appeals made to him in love by the Christians.

Hardly had this grim execution scene faded from memory than dreadful news reached them from Boyulu and Bafwasende. The tragic murder of missionaries and Europeans in these places on November 27th dashed Winnie's hopes that her colleagues were still safe. And that very moment the Simbas responsible for these atrocities were on their way to Opienge. Each village they passed they filled with terror and left panic, fear and hatred in every heart. People fled into the forest before them. On arrival at Opienge they arrested Winnie, determined on more destruction, but the local Commander released her, ransoming her and testifying openly to her goodness. So the work continued, grimly now and quietly, for the storm clouds looked very black.

It was something of a relief when General Ngalu arrived. If he proved a friend to Winnie her safety, it was thought, was assured. Everyone spoke of her faithfulness and goodness, her love for the Congolese and indentification with them. The great Ngalu cut short her case, ordering, "Don't touch her! I,

Ngalu pronounced it." Eventually he moved on to other Simba groups, inspecting, ordering, drilling.

Immediately he had gone, the Simbas took Winnie and the evangelists and threw them in prison. Three days and nights passed. Christians brought them food but could not talk to them. They sang and prayed but were summarily cuffed into silence. The dirt and lack of sanitation was appalling and if the presence of God had not been so real to them their misery would have been complete.

Ngalu heard of Winnie's imprisonment and hurried at once to release her, but meanwhile the Simbas and their president had entered her home and ransacked it, stealing *everything*. Clothes, food and radio were gone. Her radio was returned to her under Ngalu's pressure. Perhaps he was intelligent enough to value her interpretation of the English news broadcasts! Alieni and the elders pleaded with Winnie to destroy the radio, feeling sure it would land her in further trouble when Ngalu left the area again, she agreed. They beat it into smithereens on the cement floor of her house; the Simbas came in horror gathering up the scattered remnants and working on them ceaselessly to try and coax a breath of life from them, but without success.

Sunday by Sunday Winnie still preached at Opienge and many Simbas came regularly to church to hear the Word of God. Right through all the suffering the spiritual ministry of the mission was carried on.

Just before Christmas 1964 (dates were uncertain then as they had lost count), the National Army sent a plane to Boyulu to collect the remaining whites. The news reached Opienge as they were gathering in the flower-festooned church, singing hymns and rejoicing over the Saviour's birth.

The news brought joy and fear. Surely the plane would come on to Opienge for Winnie? Surely the Simbas would be mad! Deliverance seemed only a matter of hours away. What was to be done? Alieni Paul recollects: "I reminded the evangelists of our promise to protect Mademoiselle. The reminder was unnecessary. They were as concerned as I was. We decided to take her into the forest for a distance of about fifteen kilometres.

"Mademoiselle walked part of the way and we carried her the rest. She did not want to be carried but we told her, 'We have to hurry. You cannot see your way in the forest as well as we can, so we must carry you.' "

So a silent stream of people started a strange pilgrimage into the forest, deeper and deeper, winding along narrow tracks, fighting through dense undergrowth, wading along muddy streams. Circling, detouring, yet always penetrating deeper, they tried to throw off any possibility of being tracked.

Each carried a minimum: a Bible and hymn-book, a jersey and blanket and a little food. The men had weapons – spears, panga knives and bows and arrows. Every heart pounded with the tension but hopes ran high. Expectation of release made the journey easier. They were soaked through with heavy dew, scratched and torn with briers and very tired, but did not notice it. All the time their ears were stretched to hear the first murmur of an approaching plane. No one spoke and the silence seemed eerie. At last they reached the clearing where the Church had its food gardens and a halt was called.

"As we were now out of contact with happenings at Opienge *poste*," Alieni continues, "I said to the men, 'Some of us ought to go to find out what is happening. Others must remain here to protect our wives and Mademoiselle.' So the men decided who was to go back, and I and the evangelists and catechists went off to make a vast circle round the area.

"We went two by two and I was in the lead. By arrangement we kept a good distance between us so that we could give warning of possible danger ahead. We had not gone far when I saw a group of Simbas coming towards us, looking for Mademoiselle and us. With a loud voice I greeted them, so that the men coming behind heard and ran back to warn Mademoiselle."

It was a wise move on Alieni's part, as the women had heard distant voices and their hearts had almost stopped with fear.

Alieni went forward to meet the three Simbas who were armed with a gun, ammunition and spears. He discovered that one of them was one of his nephews! At the sight of him Alieni gave him something to think about.

"One day you will stand before the Holy God and He will demand an explanation of this day's affair," he said. The Simbas declared over and over again that they meant no harm. They had come to search for Winnie to return her to the village under their protection.

"With guns and spears?" asked Alieni. "You are like the soldiers who took our Lord long ago by night."

"We must take her back," they insisted.

Alieni tried to dissuade them. "She will fear you like that. Let me bring her back." But they wouldn't listen to him and refused, so he began to get angry. "Kill me instead. You won't get far except over my dead body!"

"No, no," they urged, "we didn't come to fight but in peace."

Finally the Simbas said, "We want one evangelist to go with us to find Mademoiselle; then we will kill her at the *poste*."

Alieni recalls, "I put it to the evangelists: 'Which of you will take the Simbas to Mademoiselle?' Danieli said, 'I'm ready. I'll go. If they wish to kill me, then it doesn't matter."

"So Danieli went with them but, of course, on the way he escaped and returned to us."

"Meanwhile the other evangelists had led Mademoiselle further into the forest to another place that we had already prepared for emergencies like this. We had built small temporary houses about twenty-four feet by twelve feet in secluded spots and partly stocked them with food. But always her camp bed and blankets were carried along with us on trek."

Saboni and Ana were with her all this time, as well as other friends. Once a shot broke the still air. Lying on the ground they strained every nerve to hear, but the unfriendly forest yielded no explanation. They slept uneasily under the dripping trees and a glorious array of stars in a still sky.

For several days they camped out in the forest, hungry and helpless. No plane had come and deliverance was a lost hope. Gradually news reached them of fighting, killing, villagers turning against each other, and Simba atrocities, all because of Winnie. Urgently they prayed together and Winnie, appalled at the situation, decided to hand herself over to the Simbas. She could not allow others to die in her place and she could not bear to think of others suffering while she hid. She knew she faced danger but she had a quiet confidence that her return would not involve her death.

Slowly and painfully they made their way back through the thick forests towards the food gardens. Here they met an angry mob of villagers and were shocked to see and hear much bitterness. Alieni explains what had happened: "The Simbas searching for Mademoiselle had come back after us. We did not know they were still following us . . . They had made a big detour and arrived at the village of one of our preachers called Alivazi Yoel. The Simbas had arrested Alivazi and Paul, an evangelist, while we were not far from the place where Mademoiselle had been hiding.

"Someone in the crowd called out to us, 'They have arrested two of your brethren.' I immediately called the evangelists and said, 'They have taken two of our people.'

"We ran as quickly as we could in order to try and save them. I tell you it was a fast run! When we arrived we saw two of the Simbas fighting with our two men, but our men were sitting, each on top of a Simba! Alivazi shouted when he saw us, 'Come and stand on this Simba!'

"Then as Alivazi turned, the Simba raised his gun and fired. Alivazi fell dead! Almost immediately the Simbas disappeared. We picked up the body of our brother and carried it to where Mademoiselle was hiding.

"Seeing that our lives were now in even greater danger than before, I said, 'Let each evangelist take his wife and children back to the villages. If you wish to stay there with them you may do so. If you wish to return to us here, it is your own choice.'

"So the evangelists did as I said. We were left, just Mademoiselle, Saboni, Ana, Mademoiselle's boy and myself. Then I said to Mademoiselle, 'I think it safest for me to take my children to the village. If the Simbas return here they will chase, catch and kill them.' So I left to take the children, but after I had gone the Simbas came again to search for us. I followed them and presented myself.

" 'Go and call Mademoiselle,' they said. I took them along a different path and Mademoiselle was not to be found. (Saboni had moved off with her to another spot.) So the Simbas said, 'It is an order: you must bring Mademoiselle to Opienge *poste* by 9 am Wednesday.'

"Knowing there was no alternative, we all arrived at the mission early on the Wednesday morning. We were all saddened and shaken by the death of Alivazi and the apparent hostility of his family towards Christian help. It was December 29th 1964 and we saw, shortly after 9 am, crowds of people coming to the mission – Simbas and villagers. The Simbas had come to fetch us and were fierce, deadly serious without a smile. Armed with guns, knives and sticks they approached.

" 'Where is the pastor?'

" 'Here I am.' Then in answer to a gruff, 'Come here,' I went forward. They asked for Saboni also, so he came and stood by me. They called for Mademoiselle and she stood next to us.

" 'We will go to the monument, before the State offices,' they ordered. We knew what that meant. It was the place where prisoners were executed. We had to go and they said Mademoiselle must go ahead, alone. I refused and said she must not be separated from us. We argued a long time about this but eventually she was allowed to walk between Saboni and myself. The crowds grew in number. The Simbas pushed us and made us run, but in all the confusion we did not get separated. We stuck close to Mademoiselle until we came to the offices and there we had to stand before the big crowd.

"The Simbas said, 'Pastor, you have done badly because you hid Mademoiselle in the forest, and now you have started to fight against us.'

" 'That is not the case at all,' I said. 'The fighting did not begin with us, but with you the Simbas. You came to us with anger and violence. If you had come quietly we could have settled the affair quickly. But when you came with intent to kill us we all ran and dispersed. And because we did not wish you to kill Mademoiselle out of hand, without even a hearing, we wanted to protect her in the forest.'

" 'This is your last day. You are all to die. This is your end,' they said.

"I replied, 'All right. We are ready.'

"Now before coming to the office, knowing we would not be allowed to hold conversation with one another, we arranged a foot code. The moving of the foot would not be so obvious to the crowd, who were generally occupied with looking at our faces. Any one of us could tap the other, and Mademoiselle being in the middle, would pass on the taps. One tap meant, 'Be ready for anything'; two taps, 'Pray silently with heads bowed and eyes open'; three taps, 'Get ready to meet the Lord. We shall die together'; and four taps, 'Alieni is to speak and ask why we were arrested and condemned to die'.

"Then the Simbas said, 'Before we kill them let us get ropes from the office to truss them.' This, we knew, meant experiencing the terrible '*commande*' torture. Someone struck Mademoiselle across the back with the butt of his gun but it did not seem to hurt her much.

"Then we saw a wonderful thing happen, and we can only say it was a miracle which God performed to save us from the brutal treatment intended for us. As the Simbas went to the office to fetch the ropes, the door and windows, which were closed, refused to open. The key of the door was on the table on the verandah; we could see it and so could the people. The Simbas looked for the key but could not find it. They sent to the houses where they had slept, and even to the barrier three miles away, but no one told them the key was on the table. It seems to me that God blinded the eyes of the Simbas to that key.

"Then I addressed the leader. 'If I ask permission to say something before I die, will I be granted permission?'

" 'Yes, you may speak.'

" 'Gaston,' I said, 'you are one of our tribe, a Walumbi, like Saboni and myself. Mademoiselle here is our sister. You have a wife and five children. You know the difficulty she had at their birth. You owe all your children to Mademoiselle, for if she had not been the midwife you would not have had one of them. Now you give an order to kill her. Is this good? A person like Mademoiselle at Opienge is our mother, sister, aunt and grandparent. We have become thoroughly acquainted with her. Now you want to shed her blood here at Opienge.'

"The commander then said, 'Come around the side of the house.'

"I went to him and he said, 'I have nothing against you, but I have to shout at you because of the people standing by. They must not be given to think I am friendly towards you. If you will pay me money, I will release you.'

"I said, 'All right. If that's the case I'll pay you. How much do you want?'

" 'Twenty thousand francs.'

"I returned to Mademoiselle and told her everything openly, without employing our foot code. So Saboni and I paid 5,000 francs and Mademoiselle paid 18,000 francs and we were allowed to return to the mission.

"We had a wonderful time of rejoicing. We carried Mademoiselle on our shoulders, we sang and prayed and praised the Lord for our deliverance. The Christian workers and children, shook Mademoiselle by the hand and gave her gifts, and we packed into her house talking and rejoicing until late at night."

For the next four months, January to April 1965, Winnie continued with her medical work at Opienge in relative peace. Nevertheless, four times Simbas from Bafwasende made surprise attacks on the village, seizing Winnie in the early dawn and rushing her to prison, holding her to ransom against a suspected attack by the National Army.

The prison was filthy, stinking and often crowded with people. She would stand pressed against the wall praying over them all. Each time the Simbas released her in the evening, but by then they had ransacked her house and stolen from her shamelessly.

Many nights they would come, demanding to inspect her house, insulting her, accusing her. But always the faithful Ana and Saboni stood by her and resisted them, forbidding them to molest her. Throughout those long months, through their loving care the Simbas never struck Winnie. Alieni, Noti, Leo and Danieli all stayed with her, and did everything they could to alleviate her suffering.

Alieni recalls those months: "We remained for a while at the mission compound, but almost every day there were incidents involving Mademoiselle. We decided to take her again to the forest where she could stay quiet, but they followed and found our hiding-place, This time they said Mademoiselle was to be taken to Bafwasende to be killed. We evangelists made a circle around her and refused to let them touch her. We dodged the Simbas and took her by night to another place near our own gardens. We kept her there until we knew what was happening."

Eventually the Simbas persuaded them to return, saying that no further accusations would be made against Mademoiselle, but there was a need for constant watchfulness.

"Once when they came to arrest her again they wanted to tie her with ropes and make her carry water. But we resisted them and told them, 'Brothers, if you say Mademoiselle must carry water, we the evangelists are here ready. We will draw the water.'

"This did not please them at all. We argued with them for a long time but they gave in. We had cultivated a garden for Mademoiselle with manioc, peanuts, corn and rice. We used to take her there not just to work but for her safety. The garden was a great help to her as the Simbas did not bother her there. We also arranged that someone was with her all the time.

"In May 1965 General Ngalu wanted Mademoiselle to go to his camp at Batama. "At the mission we discussed the matter thoroughly. Ngalu said, 'If Mademoiselle remains here the Simbas will continue to trouble her. If she comes with me she will be quiet.' So Mademoiselle went with Ngalu to Batama. She took medicines with her and also left a quantity to help the Simbas and ourselves. But we never had them for our use, as the Simbas stole them all."

During those troubled months the Christians had carefully divided out their medicines and stores and buried them in different parts of the station, bringing them out little by little to prevent their wholesale destruction by the rebels. It seemed that God wonderfully protected the hospital and maternity while Winnie was there. Once all the beds and mattresses were stolen for the barracks, but General Ngalu had them returned! Priscilla and three other nursing students from Nebobongo – Philbert, Ephraim and Jonah – stayed all through, helping the one trained nurse, Alexandre.

The one Dutch priest who remained, Father Strijbosch, became a close friend of Winnie's. All other Europeans had left but these two stayed, willingly offering themselves to God. They had many long talks and rejoiced together at their privilege to be considered worthy to suffer for Christ.

When General Ngalu came to collect Winnie in May he wanted her help with the medical work at Batama, midway between Bafwasende and Stanleyville on the main road, where he had his own headquarters and there was a Roman Catholic hospital and centre. He wanted her to run the hospital and maternity there for his many wounded soldiers, and care for their wives and children. Not least, he wanted her to teach English to his own children!

He arrived one sunny afternoon at about 4 pm and had tea with Winnie. Always when Ngalu was about there was a sense of peace and security, for he was a strong and able leader and would have no nonsense amongst his men. After discussing his plan with the church leaders, Winnie packed everything quickly, and next morning, after breakfast, all but one large tin trunk was stowed on Ngalu's pick-up, including table and chairs, her bed and cooking utensils.

With Winnie went her faithful house-lad Adabu Correction

and adopted son David. It was hard to leave her family, yet all felt this was the best plan. They had prayed together and sang a hymn as she left, sitting in the cab comfortably with Ngalu himself driving. Several soldiers were in the back to protect her goods.

Ngalu was faithful to his word and always respected Winnie. He gave her a room in his own house to be sure she was never molested or troubled by soldiers, and he guarded her well. He saw that she had food and did his best to provide her with extras. She worked in the hospital and maternity there and all was quiet.

Winnie had now parted from Alieni Paul. Philbert and Priscilla and Pastor Alieni stayed on at Opienge to look after the hospital and maternity and the church. The Simbas turned in fury on Alieni and Saboni because they had been Winnie's friends. They beat them up time and time again, certain that they had hidden wealth from Winnie.

Winnie was allowed to send letters to Opienge freely and to receive replies. Alieni recalls: "Mademoiselle wrote several letters to us and we wrote to her . . . In one letter to us at Opienge she said: 'Greetings to all the evangelists, the Christians and all at Opienge. If the Lord helps us we shall meet again and that will be good. Do not let down God's standard. Stand firm. And you, evangelists, be strong so that you can care for the Church of the future. If I die we shall all meet together in Heaven. But all things are in the hand of God.'

"In our opinion Mademoiselle was a very courageous person. She was more like a man than a woman in her courage. She was strong of character for preaching and for extending the work of God. Some of the Simbas repented and turned to God under her preaching and became her true friends.

"There at Ngalu's Mademoiselle had a little respite. She remained there most of 1965. Ngalu put at her disposal buildings for her medical work and she was fully occupied. One Simba who had been a school teacher found salvation through her teaching and helped her with school work.

"When the National Army began to advance in June 1966 Ngalu arranged for all to escape into the Maganga forest between Lubutu and Opienge – a very deep forest. Because of the shortage of food Mademoiselle sent her boy to Opienge to see what he could get. The Simbas urged the boy not to go back. They said, 'You will be killed.' But he went back to Mademoiselle.

"After June 1966 Ngalu tried to hand her over to the National Army, but he never succeeded. And the rumour that Mademoiselle became his wife was untrue. There was a time when the commander, adjutant, colonel, captain and all in turn tried to win her or force her into living with them. Mademoiselle wept over this and I stood between them and said that they could not touch her without killing me first. We all said the same and truly meant it. So the Simbas never touched her."

After running away from the Simbas in January 1967, Alieni had no more contact with Winnie. He was not able to emerge from the forest until March and, like the rest, had only heard intermittently that she was alive and being moved from place to place in company with the Roman Catholic priest.

Helen Roseveare continues the story. "Since June 1966, when they evacuated Batama before the approach of the National Army, they have moved from place to place in long marches through the jungle. This is Winnie's greatest difficulty. Her feet and legs are swollen and painful. She is painfully thin but mostly in good health.

"Up till January 13th 1967 Alieni stayed at the mission at Opienge and preached every Sunday. Then again he was taken prisoner and for eight days bound, hung up, beaten and almost killed; he was released for two days, then taken again and subjected to hard labour. The Simba in charge of his gang was a backslider, the son of a pastor, and he arranged Alieni's escape. So on January 25th he set off, found his wife and six children and began the long walk, hiding by day and creeping forward at night. By doubling back and dodging about like hunted animals they reached liberty on March 28th."

Alieni was able to speak of his own experiences and those of his fellow Christians at Opienge. The mission station and Church had suffered greater losses than any other WEC station. Four evangelists and one catechist had been killed and another died later. Not a building remained standing on the station, as all were demolished and the materials carried away. But the Christians had not wavered, and still stood firm determined to rebuild what was lost.

The greatest efforts to rescue Winnie were still to be made. As spring blossomed into summer in Britain new urgency stirred Christians to pray for a definite answer to their prayers.

11

THE CURTAIN LIFTS

Unevangelized Fields Mission,
Maganga, Congo
May 17th 1967

Dear Mr and Mrs Kerrigan,

Many thanks to hear your news and you to hear mine about Mlle Winnie Davies who is in the hand of Ngalu, and now I do not know her news.

I was captured by Ngalu August 10th 1966 because I was the first against the Revolution in Baego. On arriving at Batama, without the help of our sister Mlle, I would have been killed at that time and at that date. I was imprisoned until the eleventh month.

Ngalu did not want me to return to Baego and said that I would teach people bad teaching. Then he forced me to join the rebels and sent me to Opienge on November 22nd 1966. We were with Mlle and we helped each other very much. When we heard that the National Army had arrived at the Tsoppo River my thoughts and the thoughts of others were to hide Mlle and when the NA arrived we would go out to them.

When they sent me to Opienge, after two weeks I fled with a school teacher who was also a prisoner. We reached Bafwasende in the fourth month and we left Mlle at Batama. But I have heard news of Mlle. In April 1967 I heard she was well, and also the Roman Catholic Father. Another word I heard was that they stole Mlle's clothes and that she was weaker in body than when we left her . . .

This letter from a Congolese Christian, Elia Joseph Mayangbo, served to confirm reports that Winnie was physically weaker, and that her European companion in captivity was a Roman Catholic priest.

Father Alphons Strijbosch is the "Roman Catholic Father" mentioned in the letter. Having worked at Opienge through the rebellion, he joined Winnie at Batama in August 1966 at Ngalu's invitation. It is he who takes up the story for us, lifting the curtain of silence over those months of captivity and flight from the National Army.

I met Father Alphons in his beautiful native village of Erp, Holland. Forty-seven years of age, of stocky build with well-trimmed beard and thin greying hair, he looked comparatively fit considering the three years he had spent under rebel rule. He had been liberated only seven weeks when I saw him and as we shook hands the priest looked around, then up at the sky and said, "It is wonderful to be free. How Miss Davies and I used to envy the birds and monkeys in the jungle. For days on end we did not see the sun because of the dense forest growth; it was dark, damp and cold. We were not able to do as we wished and go where we wanted to go. Now I feel like a bird liberated from his cage."

We chatted as we walked to meet his eighty-year-old father and married sister, at whose home he was staying during his recuperation and reorientation. He had been in the Congo for twenty years. I noticed he was a little nervous of the traffic and he smiled as he said, "I wonder if I shall ever become sufficiently accustomed to be able to ride a bicycle in all this."

When we had settled into comfortable armchairs he sat for a time deep in thought.

"I do not find it easy to recall everything that happened during the occupation," he explained. "I would have to sit long and think deeply. I was not able to make any notes, you see. And sometimes I feel so glad it is all over that I do not care to think back over it at all."

Remembering the first days of the takeover at Opienge by the Simbas in August 1964, Father Alphons mentioned the tension and state of "nerves" which prevailed. There was roughly a mile between his station and Winnie's and periodically he went across to see how she was faring. "It was bad enough for me, a man, to live in that awful atmosphere. It was much worse for her, a woman. We had very friendly relations but did not meet more than once a month, so that we would not be suspected of political intrigue.

"Almost daily there were incidents and difficulties. It made Mademoiselle nervous and fearful. She did not come out of the compound to the motor road, but remained in her house or in the maternity with the teachers or the women. She helped the women prepare meals and went with them to their gardens. But often the Simbas came to the compound and roughly demanded anything they fancied. In that way her stocks of medicines, sugar, salt, etc., were quickly depleted.

"One day the commander called us both and put us in prison. We remained there the whole day. Towards evening Mademoiselle was returned to her mission because she was needed for a maternity case. Some weeks later we were called for again. When I arrived at the *poste* I found Mademoiselle sitting on the ground near the flagpost. We had to listen to a speech in which we were terribly maligned and insulted. They had the idea that we had power to call planes, so we were told that if a plane passed that way we should be killed.

"We were put in the prison again, and strangely enough, within about fifteen minutes a plane was heard. Mademoiselle was greatly distressed and we both wondered what the Simbas would do to us, but nothing happened. We were kept in the cell: a small dark room. Our companions were women who practised witchcraft, who had been accused of doing harm through the power of the evil spirits by whom they were supposed to be possessed. After two days we were released.

"It was at that time the Christian workers took Mademoiselle away into the forest to hide and protect her from the rebels. I cannot speak too highly of those workers; they were splendid men who could be trusted.

"We had to put up with a lot of harsh treatment. One of the

Simba officers, a Yakusu from Banyema, was very hard on me. He came for loads of rice but sent for me and made me lie full length on the ground. He put his rifle in my stomach, his feet on my head and said, 'Tomorrow, if I don't see Ngalu I shall kill you.' He let me lie for a while, then added, 'Get up. Take off your shoes and wait here until Mademoiselle arrives; then you will both draw water for me.'

"When Mademoiselle arrived the Simbas produced a huge water-drum slung on a pole. They placed the pole on her shoulder and mine, with the drum swinging between us, then ordered us to run barefoot to the spring which was at the bottom of a steep incline. The sharp stones cut painfully into our feet, causing us to stumble; after the first journey we had to empty the water into large containers and go back again to the spring.

"By the time we had done two trips Mademoiselle was crying with pain and fatigue. She kept repeating '*Mungu Baba, Mungu Baba!*' (Oh, Heavenly Father!) – a phrase which was often on her lips. Finally we were told to return to our respective missions."

Father Strijbosch also told of an occasion when he was made to stand with a mulatto to be executed. The Simba's finger was on the trigger when another Simba put his hand on the gun and prevented the shot. The priest was then told to show the Simbas where the mission money was kept. He led the way to the Catholic mission and showed them where the money was hidden. They helped themselves to the whole lot. They had already taken his car and camionnette, but they could not take his truck because the engine was at Stanleyville for repairs!

"Just after November 24th," he continues, "(that was the day the Belgian paratroopers rescued the whites at Stanleyville) two groups of Simbas came to seek for me at the mission. They stood at a distance calling me out to them. I asked them what they wanted but they would not reply. Then I saw they were all armed with spears, guns and sticks.

"I wondered what was going to happen, for it looked dangerous. Fear gripped me. I decided to run into the plantation and hide but they caught up with me, beating me with all the weapons they had. My sun helmet was completely smashed. I was thrown to the ground and my hands were tied. They were going to give me the *commande* torture, but someone arrived breathlessly with a message from the official to say that I should not be given this horrible trussing and beating.

"The ropes were loosened and I was taken to the official.

" 'Why did you run away?' he asked.

" 'If you want me, come and fetch me yourself and do not send a pack of roughs again to take me by force. I ran because I was afraid of what they might do to me.'

"Finally he told me to open the rooms and cupboards in my house. He took my radio and anything else he fancied, then said, 'Wash yourself, then go to Mademoiselle for treatment for your wounds.'

"That was the first time I was beaten, but on many later occasions I had to go to Mademoiselle for treatment of wounds received as a result of being beaten. Mademoiselle was never beaten severely but I do know she was once or twice struck across the back with the butt of a gun. We were very fortunate not to be subjected to the full *commande* treatment. It was given to blacks as well as whites. At Bafwasende, later on, I saw two Congolese killed in that terrible fashion. One was a Babari policeman and the other a member of the Partie Nationale Populaire. The latter's body was put in the boot of a car and then thrown into the river."

A month after the massacre at Boyulu and Bafwasende, on the last day of 1964, a rebel official came to interview Winnie and the priest. The following day Father Strijbosch was taken by truck to Bafwasende and kept there for seventeen days. On one of the walls of the Roman Catholic dwelling he passed he saw written in Swahili, "We have gone. Goodbye. We pray for you." Then followed the names of the priests, seven of whom had been killed. The sisters, together with the Boyulu women missionaries, had been saved. On his return to Opienge, Father Strijbosch called to see Winnie and told her the news of the writing on the wall and the fate of the priests. Their hearts were deeply stirred as they realized afresh their own danger.

In May 1965 Ngalu came to fetch Winnie and the priest was present at her departure. "The day Ngalu came to take Mademoiselle to his camp at Batama I remember she went crying to the truck. I talked with her and tried to reassure her, but she felt very deeply that she was being taken from her people.

" 'It will probably be better for you at Batama,' I said. 'The Simbas will not be allowed to trouble you. Besides, one must submit to the will of God in such matters.' She was soon calm after that and even seemed happy to be going. She was able to take some personal belongings with her in the truck. The road at that time was still usable.

"Mademoiselle remained at Batama from May 1965 until June 1966; then they moved to another camp a few kilometres from the road. She continued with her medical work and also took morning and evening services in the chapel, as Ngalu had given permission for this.

"The other leader, who was under Ngalu, was against Mademoiselle having so much liberty. He was Dominique Babu, State Defence Minister in pre-revolution days, a professed atheist who had studied four years in France and six months in Moscow and Peking. Despite his claim to superior learning he was a polygamist with at least thirteen wives.

"Mademoiselle still had her house-boy with her at Batama. He was a faithful lad who had been with her for some years and would not leave her. Also she still had David, the child she had cared for since he was a baby.

"The next time we met was in August 1966 when I was called to Ngalu's camp near Batama. Until then I had been with the Director of the Political Bureau; now this minister was promoted Colonel and Ngalu became General. At Batama I found the Roman Catholic church had been destroyed; all that remained was the bell. I asked the Simbas why they had done this and they said, 'We do it in order to prevent people looting.'!

"From that time I lived in the same compound as Mademoiselle, she in one hut and I in another about two hundred metres away. We were free to talk to one another and when we did not want the Africans to know what we were talking about we used English! Mademoiselle had a cat then, of which she was very fond, but later it ran away and became wild probably through lack of food. Ngalu gave her a parrot which was called 'Chako' and this also gave her some entertainment.

"We shared a great deal in our mutual poverty. We cultivated a maize garden for ourselves and often had our meals together. If she had food she would send for me to come and share it. The food usually consisted of plantains, manioc leaves (a kind of spinach), and sometimes a piece of rotting, smelly meat from which we had to chase away the flies." The priest laughed as he remembered.

"Another source of entertainment was a radio that Mademoiselle was given, but she had to return it later as it belonged to one of the Simba officials. To fill my time I was ordered to teach English and Latin to Ngalu's children. One day Ngalu produced a book on algebra and told me to teach that to his children as well. I wondered where he had looted the book from. He was eager that his children should be educated in order that they should get on in the world."

Father Strijbosch recalls that in August or September 1966 Winnie became gravely ill with malaria. The Congolese male nurses found one or two anti-malaria tablets for her and the Father also gave her a couple of Atebrine tablets from the eight or ten he had left. He had previously had about two thousand of these tablets but the Simbas had relieved him of them.

Winnie was very feeble, terribly thin, and obviously very weak for she said to Father Strijbosch one morning, "I think I shall die tonight." But she recovered, although weakened by her illness.

"About October 1966 the National Army must have learned the whereabout of the Simbas, for the bombardments began." The priest continues, "Each day we had to escape into the forest, returning in the evening. On one occasion five planes came over. Life became insupportable, so Ngalu decided to move to Camp Lumumba, ten kilometres away. The real name was Camp Lomboya but we were not allowed to call it that, in order to hide its exact location.

"I remember Mademoiselle did not appreciate the NA's attempts to catch the rebels. She said to me, 'It is a pity that the NA encircle us with their planes for I have no desire to walk this distance; I am so weak!' But a week later we had to go. On the way Mademoiselle complained that she could not keep up, so she was allowed to rest for the night in a shack with a Simba guard sleeping outside. I also remember how she arrived next day, leaning on her stick and incredibly dirty. It had been a filthy journey with plenty of mud. We sank up to our knees in the mud; then, in extricating our legs, our shoes would remain embedded, necessitating a long arm plunge to rescue them. You can imagine our dirty condition!

"On some of the marches we were ordered to walk backwards so that our footprints would deceive any followers. We also had to learn to drop leaves and fronds as directives on side paths so as to lead pursuers on to wrong trails.

"It is no wonder that we found these journeys trying, and we were not the only ones. The Congolese women, carrying loads, could hardly keep up. One woman, in desperation, abandoned her child. Some Simba soldiers came across the child in the bush and carried it on their shoulders to the next stopping place.

"Besides these forced marches food was an increasing problem. At one time we had as many as three to four deaths daily owing to hunger, and many of the natives suffered from beri-beri. There were two great difficulties. We had to hide from the planes and bombardments, and yet we had to search for food. It was like playing hide and seek, but this game was a desperately serious one.

"Each time we moved camp it was to go further into the forest and there it was increasingly difficult to find food. We learnt to recognize certain edible plants and mushrooms and we made a salad out of the tender sprouts of a leaf that the Africans use for roofing their houses. Sometimes when we shuddered at some of the African dishes (a fat mother ant three or four inches long, a certain type of caterpillar, and worse) we would laugh and say, 'There is no difference between the stomach of a black man and a white man, so what is good for one must be good for the other!' We found this attitude enabled us to eat the most unpalatable foods but then, when hunger really gets you, you'll eat anything.

"There was such a demand for food that the plantains were not allowed to ripen. When we did succeed in getting some they were usually small and immature. Sometimes we had rice and a little palm oil but we had to pound the rice paddy ourselves. Very rarely we were given a few peanuts. Once the Simbas killed a buffalo and another beast, and that was good for us because we were always given a small piece of meat after the kill. We had to use this sparingly to make it last two or three days. To cook the food we lit a fire with either a burning faggot that we carried with us or a light borrowed from one of the women's fires. Ngalu had matches but we did not.

"Sometimes fighting broke out between the Simbas and villagers. Bloodshed was common. Ngalu killed many people, even mothers with children in their arms. The Simbas would go off on a blood-hunt, knocking on doors and shouting '*Mutoke inje*' (Come outside). If the people emerged the Simbas would say, 'You've come out because you thought we were the NA. You are against the new regime so you must die.' If the villagers did not emerge they were shot anyway for not obeying the order!"

At Camp Lumumba Winnie was given a hut by one of the Christians but was moved again after a week. This time she was given a house which had been erected for General Ngalu. He and his family had not yet arrived at camp. She still had a camp bed, blankets, mattress and a small valise. Also she had kept two Bibles, one Swahili and the other English. "Later in 1967," Father Strijbosch adds, "Ngalu asked her for her Swahili Bible and me for my rosary. I still had my little book of prayers. I remember an African woman always carried Mademoiselle's

Bible and her bundle of two or three bed sheets and one blanket for her."

If conditions had been bad, they were to get far worse as the National Army intensified its efforts to catch the rebels. Father Strijbosch continues: "I believe we must have stayed at Camp Lumumba until about the end of October 1966. The National Army was advancing on the main road and we could hear the mortars near Batama. There was a fear that the soldiers might come right into the forest so we had to move again, about another ten kilometres farther into the forest. It was only a temporary camp and we remained there about one week, during which time Mademoiselle lived with Ngalu's wives.

"It was getting extremely difficult to find food and we were often hungry now. There were times when we had absolutely nothing to cook. In fact, I ate only when someone found a bit of food and invited me to join in. If I wasn't called – or called and didn't run to it – I had nothing at all! I soon realized how easily you can starve to death in the forest. We depended on the goodwill of the Simbas to keep us alive. We still had a few utensils, knives, forks and pots, so when we had food we ate from the pots using the lids as plates.

"The Africans went hungry too. The Simbas found one woman boiling the flesh of her own child! Whether the child had died from natural causes or had been killed I do not know, nor do I remember how the case was decided.

"Next we had to move another ten or fifteen kilometres to Camp Omeka and here Mademoiselle was again taken seriously ill. There was a male nurse in the camp but Mademoiselle was too ill to go across to him for treatment. She had to be carried in a sort of rough carrying chair which they strung up for her. She was given a hut by one of Ngalu's officers not far from Ngalu's house, and there she rested and found some food. I think she remained there for two-and-a-half to three weeks."

It was now December 1966. Winnie was further weakened by illness and the continued physical hardship, which showed no sign of letting up.

"One morning Mademoiselle had sent her house-boy to the road to look for food when suddenly the order came to move on. Mademoiselle went ahead of me because she had succeeded in finding someone to carry some of her things. This was because the Simbas the previous night had had a roll-call and allocated certain people to carry luggage. But two men failed to turn up, which meant that half of Mademoiselle's goods and mine remained behind. Fortunately, the baggage arrived later. Mademoiselle had some manioc in her trunk, but on opening it found that the manioc was rotten and had to be thrown away.

"I caught up with Mademoiselle at the first stop; she was trying to rest. She gave me three plantains. She was indeed good and generous, always helping me readily. When the time came to continue the journey she had great difficulty, as we had three days' steady marching up and down hill, through mud, across streams and along narrow paths. It had been raining, and 'after rain' falling from the trees continued for a long time until we were drenched to the skin and very cold.

"The first day had not been so very bad but the second day tried me greatly and I thought, 'Mademoiselle will never make it.' And so it proved. She was not able to keep up and lodged somewhere en route. Fortunately a Simba official and I had passed her, and he had realized she was too weak to make the journey and left a Simba there with her. She managed to find some manioc flour and rice husks after somebody's winnowing. She made a kind of paste for us to eat and said, 'There will be vitamins left in the husks, so we must eat it.' "

Father Strijbosch commented here that though food was an extreme problem, thirst was a far greater trial. It became unbearable and they had to drink from whatever source they could find. There were, of course, no amenities for boiling water for drinking, but then, as there was very little hope of rescue and life, why should they fear to drink contaminated water? He and Winnie would quote the African proverb "*Maiti haigopi saanda*" (The corpse does not fear the coffin)!

"After about three or four days' marching Mademoiselle

arrived at Camp Ngalu and was given a hut in the temporary part of the camp. Ngalu was still at Camp Omeka, where he remained for another month.

"Mademoiselle was moved to the other end of the clearing after about a week. Here the Simbas had already begun to build a permanent camp and she was able to stay in Ngalu's house, as he had not arrived. She received her ration of rice and dried manioc regularly and sometimes was able to exchange a little for some fish. We were near the river, so many of the Simbas went fishing. David also went fishing occasionally, for he could go alone without a Simba guard. I had no house-boy or helper so I learned to prepare my own food. Also I learned that if I gave my paddy to a Simba to pound for me, I would receive only half the rice! The rest would be in his stomach! I could not afford this so I did my own work, extracting oil from the palm nuts, shredding and boiling manioc leaves, preparing and cooking manioc and plantains. We had to do this in order to live.

"But before long we once again had some days of desperate hunger. Mademoiselle even went pleading to the Colonel and finally received a little food. She was very weak at the time, and had great difficulty in climbing the hill back to her part of the camp when she occasionally came across to the temporary part. The whole terrain was very hilly and the plastic shoes she was wearing were cracked in places. Someone had given them to her and she had tried to mend them with wire.

"I was more fortunate with footwear. Just before those long marches my shoes wore out, so a Simba lent me his boots. My feet are size seven and his boots were size eight. With the good pairs of socks I had these boots were a wonderful help. The Simba who gave them to me ran away and gave himself up to the National Army, so I was able to keep them!" The priest chuckled as he remembered the incident. "Later on the boots became very broken and I had to tie them together with vine strings cut from the forest, and walking then became increasingly difficult.

"Mademoiselle had lots of wounds and scratches. Her sandals

and shoes were the open kind, so her feet were unprotected from thorns and sharp undergrowth. We had to force our way through uncut vegetation, suffering greatly from the backlash of rough branches and the rasp-like leaves which are common in the jungle. Often we were cut across the face and neck, when we were hurrying to keep up with the Simbas; we did not seem to mind these scratches, but afterwards we were in agony. Beside the scratches Mademoiselle had many infected bites which she cleansed with hot water when she could. And even worse than that was a painful abcess caused by a dirty needle used by an African nurse to inject her when she was ill. Added to all this we had bouts of dysentery, then constipation, and were the prey of insects. Once we were attacked by a swarm of bees and several times we found elephant ticks enjoying a meal at our expense. Living in the open encouraged this general weakening of our bodily resistance. On some of these forced marches we had to sleep under the sky; in the morning we could wring water out of our blankets, from the dew or the rain.

"At Camp Ngalu, Mademoiselle was eventually given an empty food storehouse, a mud hut, and two weeks later I joined her. She was in the completed part of the house with David and her house-boy, while I was given the verandah, which had one end closed with plaited leaves and the other end completely open to the elements. It was an unfortunate arrangement, for every time it rained my mattress got wet. I managed to cover most of the open section with large leaves, making it more secure from the rain and wind.

"I remember that while she was in the food hut Mademoiselle was able to attend to the pregnant wife of the officer who had passed her on the journey to Camp Ngalu. He was the Ordnance officer. I remember, too, that we were there under the one roof from January to Easter 1967. Having my prayer-book helped me to remember such dates, for there are prayers in the book up to 1990 for various religious festivals. I kept the prayer days and well remember Easter 1967, for it was then I asked to become instructor of Ngalu's little school.

"We were separated when Mademoiselle was moved to a hut behind the hill in the camp. It had been used by a Simba. From this hut she sent her house-boy to look for food and he returned with three chickens!

"On Easter Monday 1967 there was another scare and we were made to hurriedly escape from the camp, walking for about an hour. Mademoiselle was a bit ahead of me, but we camped together for two or three days. During that time the General came and joined us while on a hunting trip. He knew we needed food and was hunting buffalo. We suddenly heard shooting while he was away, but he returned empty-handed. We were told that while returning in a canoe with his kill – one buffalo – he had been attacked by NA soldiers. Leaving the meat in the canoe he had jumped into the water and escaped swimming. Two Simbas were killed in the incident and two, besides the General, were saved. On his return to the camp Ngalu turned to Mademoiselle and said, 'You can see I also am a man of God, otherwise God would not have allowed me to escape from the NA soldiers!' "

Father Strijbosch went on to describe the conditions and morale of the Simbas as they fled from the National Army. The party was a small one by this time because of the deaths from hunger and desertions due to the general lack of confidence. The fifty people left, ten men and forty women, seemed to have little contact with other Simbas. There were many thousands of rebels in the forest but little liaison between them. This was often because transmitters had ceased to function through lack of diesel oil. The Simbas tried to keep their radio batteries working by making acid from banana skins but this was not very successful. Generally speaking the regime had degenerated into scattered packs of guerilla bandits constantly hounded by the NA and constantly on the move, without any overall plan of action.

"During those precarious days Mademoiselle and I were together all the time. The General insisted on this because he always wanted to know just where we were. At the camp in the forest that night I borrowed a panga knife from a Simba and cut sticks with which to make bed frames. One frame for Mademoiselle was put at one end of the hut and one for me at the other end. Then we gathered dry leaves for mattresses. All through the night we kept a big fire burning on the floor between our beds. An armed Simba never moved from the door.

"Mademoiselle was terribly tired when we arrived at that stopping place. She just flung herself down on the leaves on the ground and lay there for a long time before she went in search of firewood for our fire.

"The women were good to Mademoiselle. They willingly gave her anything she required and were particularly helpful in lending their cooking utensils. She had, of course, made very many friends through her maternity work. Of the forty women in the camp, ten were Ngalu's 'wives'.

"Hunger still stalked us. We shared every bit of food we succeeded in finding. Mademoiselle was always so good in this way. And I learnt that it is easy to share food when you have plenty but not so easy when you are desperately hungry and have only a few teaspoonfuls of rice left. I can laugh now as I look back but I know we did not laugh then.

"Suddenly, ten days after Pentecost, we were hurried from the camp to a more protected spot because the National Army had begun to attack. The Simbas had reported seeing soldiers at the 206 Km barrier on the Route Ituri. That report came through at about 8 pm and we had to move that same evening. Instead of lamps we carried burning faggots, blowing them periodically to keep them alight. The going was difficult and we stumbled over roots, hurting our feet as we went. As usual Mademoiselle was about fifteen minutes ahead of me with the women and children but we met later in the same hut. She was again exhausted and lay on a grass mat. I sat all night on a hard 'chair', the two-stick kind that the pygmies made which are most uncomfortable during the day and a torture during the night. Sleep was out of the question! All night we were protected, if that is the word, by a Simba with a spear.

"Next morning at about 6 am we heard firing. We had to leave immediately and for four hours struggled through thick jungle, the Simbas cutting a way with their long panga knives. After four days we returned to camp, hearing that the NA had withdrawn. Ngalu had not fled with us but had hidden not far from the camp, and we had to return at his command.

"For about ten days we remained there; then, through the scouts that Ngalu had sent out in several directions, came another warning. Again we had to take to the forest after dark. Mademoiselle was well ahead of me and had taken another path. I heard the Colonel shout, 'Do not stop. Continue in the dark.' And we did, for two hours! A terrible journey. Finally we lodged somewhere in an awful place full of stinging gnats. I had a mosquito net but it was useless against the tiny creatures, so I rolled myself up in my blanket, head and all.

"Fortunately Mademoiselle had gone with Ngalu's family. I met up with her three days later. She was in a little shelter with a bed of leaves and a fire on the ground. On seeing me she immediately gave me a little hard boiled rice, which I cut with a knife as it was solid. I was glad to have it, but you cannot eat much of it at a time as it swells in the stomach. We camped there until the next day.

"Meanwhile I had some difficulty with the General. He had lost contact with his wives and children, so he poured his wrath on me. In great anger he accused me of sending someone to call the soldiers to liberate us. (I had no means of doing this even if I had wanted to.)

" '*Utakufa leo, hakuna ubishi,*' (You will die today, without a doubt) he shouted. I was led away to be killed.

"Suddenly the General yelled at us, calling me back. We talked and I swore to him that I knew nothing about anyone going to call the soldiers. He said he intended killing me because of something he had been told. He said I had touched his gun that evening when the stinging gnats had been so troublesome. As I had not even seen his gun, it seemed to me someone was seeking to make trouble for me. Finally he turned to Mademoiselle, who had heard everything.

" 'Tell the priest not to touch my gun or he will certainly die,' he commanded, and she obeyed.

"Next day there was yet another forced march. For food we had a little rice, made up in leaf packets in the shape of cylinders. Mademoiselle and I shared a cylinder and a piece of dried fish. But those days of forced marching were inhuman. We simply had to keep going for six or seven hours a day without sitting. At the most we were allowed to stand for three or four minutes to straighten our breaking backs. The Simbas refused to let us sit.

" 'If you sit, your muscles will contract and you will be unable to go on,' they said.

"This grim ordeal did not help Mademoiselle. Her legs now became excessively swollen. For a long time she had suffered from palpitations and I remember her saying that her pulse rate was a hundred and fifty. She found the physical strain increasingly difficult to bear. But, in spite of this, on the second day of marching she successfully delivered one of the women of a baby, without medicines or instruments – not even a pair of scissors."

. . .

On May 27th Strijbosch and his Simba guard, an old man, lost their way in a maze of buffalo and elephant paths. He could not keep up any longer and he knew that Winnie must be exhausted, for he himself had fallen twice through faintness. He and his guard, having crossed two rivers, dared to risk a few minutes' pause to eat a little food. As they pushed on they realized that they had been going in a circle, for they recognized the path as one which the fleeing Simbas had already taken.

Almost immediately the priest saw Winnie lying at the side of the path. She looked just as he had seen her on other occasions, flat out on her back and thoroughly spent. But on coming nearer he was shocked to see wounds above her eyes and a cut on her throat. The blood was fresh and still trickling from the scars and he realized she could not have been dead more than fifteen to twenty minutes.

Too dazed to think properly, he turned away. Suddenly it dawned on him that if they had killed Winnie they would certainly kill him. They had always said, "If we come to killing the whites, you will be the first and Mademoiselle will be the last." And he remembered the order that had been given that morning: "Stragglers will be killed, as we are leaving no one for the NA to collect behind us." Winnie had heard the order and had murmured "That includes me." Realizing now the full danger he was in, Father Strijbosch slung his bundle off his shoulder to the ground. Automatically he checked through his few possessions, then repacked them. They seemed to weigh like solid lead on his back. He stood for a minute, uttered a prayer, then took his stick and trudged forward.

Barely five hundred yards farther on he saw three forms appear from the jungle. They were soldiers with raised guns. Startled, he thought, "This is the end. Ngalu has sent these men to kill me for failing to keep up."

Quickly he crossed himself and threw up his arms.

"Are you the Roman Catholic priest?" one of the soldiers shouted.

"I am."

"We are the National Army. You are rescued!"

What a moment! Bewildered, he stared blankly at the soldiers. Could it be true at long last? But oh, if only they had arrived just twenty minutes earlier!

Not knowing whether to laugh or cry he approached his liberators. He was so tired physically and mentally that he was stunned by the sudden and incredible turn of events. In his dazed state it never occurred to him to return to Winnie's body, to collect anything at all to verify his report to consuls and others. In any case there was not much he could have brought, except perhaps a snippet of her dress, the only one she now possessed. The Simbas had stolen everything else, including her watch and spectacles.

The soldiers had seen Winnie's body, but were concerned to get the priest to safety as soon as possible. To do this they had to walk sixty-five miles through the jungle, sleeping three or four nights on the way. Reaching the motor road they were able to transmit the news of Winnie's death and the priest's deliverance to the authorities.

A band of Congolese Red Cross workers went to meet the priest as he arrived at the road, and receiving details of the route they walked the sixty-five miles to search for the body. Valiantly they struggled back with their burden in a zinc metal coffin, and reached Km 206 on the Route Ituri. From there the body was taken to Kisangani (Stanleyville) where permission was granted for the interment to be made at the edge of the common grave where the mass burial had taken place of the whites murdered at Kisangani on November 27th 1964.

. . .

The funeral took place on June 16th 1967. The Kerrigans, recipients of the letter that opened this chapter, sent this report.

"Yesterday we laid Miss Winifred Davies to rest in the same cemetery and in the same grave as Mr Cyril Taylor and Miss Muriel Harman, her fellow missionaries, who with some thirty Roman Catholic priests and nuns were martyred in 1964.

"In the morning we went to the Botanical Gardens to order flowers. When we went to collect and pay for them the Congolese gardeners told us there was nothing to pay. It was their tribute to the Mademoiselle who had given her life for their country. They had arranged three beautiful sprays of flowers: frangipani, jasmine, tuberoses and evergreens – a real work of art.

"At 3 pm we gathered in the Baptist Missionary Society church for the service conducted by Pastor Mokili François. The casket was already there. The Governor of Kisangani was present, also General Tshinyama, Colonel Zongi and some thirty soldiers of the National Army who had composed the rescue party. Colonel Brook Fox, the British Military Attaché from Kisangani, represented the British Ambassador. Congolese pastors, evangelists, teachers, Christians, missionaries,

Roman Catholic priests and nuns, and Europeans from the town were present to pay tribute to a devoted servant of the Lord.

"The BMS church choir sang quietly and reverently, in French, a hymn which portrayed the everlasting happiness of those in Heaven. During the service we all sang "Peace, perfect peace' and 'Shall we gather at the River?'. In Lingala we sang 'We shall gather in Heaven'. Pastor Asani, the Rev. George Kerrigan and Colonel Brook Fox paid tributes and gave thanks for Winnie's life and witness. Pastor Bo Martin read the Scriptures and gave the message. Major Lesserre of the Salvation Army prayed.

"At the close of the service we filed out of the church to make our way to the cemetery. Eighteen or more cars, jeeps and trucks followed the cortège. As we slowly passed the Roman Catholic cathedral the bell rang and then tolled. Groups of people stood quietly as we passed and soldiers and police stood to attention and saluted.

"At the cemetery the choir led the way to the graveside singing 'My Jesus I love Thee, I know Thou art mine'. The Rev. David Claxton conducted the burial service. We sang 'Blessed Assurance' and the casket was lowered gently into the grave at 5 pm, in sight of the Congo River. Two lovely wreaths from the Governor and General Tshinyama were laid, then a beautiful spray from the Roman Catholic sisters, and finally one from Winnie's friends at Opienge."

In Caxton Hall, London, on the same day, June 16th, 1967, a Service of Remembrance and Thanksgiving was held. The International Secretary of the Worldwide Evangelization Crusade gave the Thanksgiving Address, basing his message on Paul's words in Philippians 1 : 20: "According to my earnest expectation and my hope, that in nothing I shall be ashamed, but that with all boldness, as always, so now also Christ shall be magnified in my body, whether it be by life, or by death." This was Winnie's favourite text and she quoted it to her missionary colleagues before leaving for the last time for the Congo.

Mr Moules commented: "Paul was an intense personality, and

his language was similarly highly powered. What he says in its fullest meaning is 'I am concentrating on watching Christ, so that I shall not be ashamed, but full of courage as He draws back the curtain on my life to reveal Himself by my life or by my death.' We may compare this to the mechanics of the stage, of the theatre, of drawing back the curtain in order that the players and cast may be revealed on the stage.

"I believe Winnie, too, was an intense personality. Her conviction of what she knew to be the mind of the Lord could at times be embarrassing to her missionary colleagues. I am sure this was because of the dynamic pressure that she brought to bear on the matters that were under consideration. Therefore, I am not surprised that Winnie found this was the text that could portray her inner feeling and recommissioning in Christ as she faced again the Congo. So she looked with intense concentration into the future – and little did she know what God was going to do to lift the curtain of life to reveal Himself. God appointed Judas to Jesus. God appointed General Ngalu to Winnie . . . Now we see in this broken life the curtain fully drawn back. We do not see Winnie – we see the Lord. Christ alone is revealed. It was from Him came the stream of courage, fortitude, and fulfilment of duty. Winnie has gone, Christ remains, central and glorious in this broken life."